MEETING THE NEED FOR
Psychosocial Care in Young Adults With Cancer

By Anne Katz, PhD, RN, FAAN

Oncology Nursing Society
Pittsburgh, Pennsylvania

ONS Publications Department

Executive Director, Professional Practice and Programs: Elizabeth Wertz Evans, PhD, RN, MPM, CPHQ, CPHIMS, FHIMSS, FACMPE
Publisher and Director of Publications: William A. Tony, BA, CQIA
Managing Editor: Lisa M. George, BA
Assistant Managing Editor: Amy Nicoletti, BA, JD
Acquisitions Editor: John Zaphyr, BA, MEd
Copy Editor: Vanessa Kattouf, BA
Graphic Designer: Dany Sjoen
Editorial Assistant: Judy Holmes

Library of Congress Cataloging-in-Publication Data

Katz, Anne (Anne Jennifer), 1958-, author.
  Meeting the need for psychosocial care in young adults with cancer / by Anne Katz.
     p. ; cm.
  Includes bibliographical references.
  ISBN 978-1-935864-64-6
  I. Title.
  [DNLM: 1. Health Services Needs and Demand. 2. Neoplasms–psychology. 3. Young Adult–psychology.
QZ 200]
  RC271.M4
  616.99'40651–dc23

                                                                                    2015009188

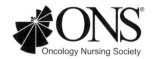

Integrity • Innovation • Stewardship • Advocacy • Excellence • Inclusiveness

As always, with gratitude to Alan for a keen eye and an open heart
And to Samuel Morris Klein, may you never be in need of any of this

Disclosure

Editors and authors of books and guidelines provided by the Oncology Nursing Society are expected to disclose to the readers any significant financial interest or other relationships with the manufacturer(s) of any commercial products.

A vested interest may be considered to exist if a contributor is affiliated with or has a financial interest in commercial organizations that may have a direct or indirect interest in the subject matter. A "financial interest" may include, but is not limited to, being a shareholder in the organization; being an employee of the commercial organization; serving on an organization's speakers bureau; or receiving research from the organization. An "affiliation" may be holding a position on an advisory board or some other role of benefit to the commercial organization. Vested interest statements appear in the front matter for each publication.

Contributors are expected to disclose any unlabeled or investigational use of products discussed in their content. This information is acknowledged solely for the information of the readers.

The author provided the following disclosure and vested interest information:

The author had no relevant information to disclose.

Contents

CHAPTER 1
Introduction

What do we know about the psychosocial needs of young adults with cancer? And are they different from those of other cancer survivors? The answers are simply "a little" for the first question and "a lot" for the second. Young adults have traditionally fallen between the two worlds of pediatric and adult cancer. However, young adults are a unique population with developmental tasks and life experiences that are different from those in other life stages.

This book will describe what is known about the psychosocial needs of young adults with cancer, mostly from the perspective of descriptive studies. How to help young adults face and overcome the challenges of cancer at this stage of life will also be addressed. The audience for this book is members of the multidisciplinary team who provide medical, nursing, and psychosocial care for these young people. The goal is for these teams to provide the best possible care for young adult cancer survivors—care that is comprehensive, and evidence based and takes into account their unique needs and stage of life. This is the least of what they deserve.

Emerging and Young Adulthood

Jeffrey Arnett (2011) is the foremost authority on the stage of life that he coined *emerging adulthood*—the ages between 18 and 24. The rationale behind this term is that over the past 50 years, the years between adolescence and young adulthood have taken on some unique characteristics that are not accurately reflected in adolescence (up to age 18) and young adulthood (age 25–45). Today, individuals engage in college education for extended periods, delay marriage and childbearing, and may live in their parents' homes until their early 30s. Arnett (2011) noted that these years have key characteristics of
• Identity exploration

- Instability
- Self-focus
- Feeling "in-between"
- The age of possibilities.

It is in this stage of life that individuals explore their personal identities—whom they choose to love and what they choose to do for work. These judgments are based on their interests and preferences. This is a time of instability because inherent in the many choices is a change in partners, living arrangements, or educational direction. It is also a stage that is focused on the self because at this age, people have few responsibilities and obligations and are able to think only about what they want or need. At this stage, individuals feel as though they are in between adolescence and young adulthood. It is also the age of possibilities because of the hope and belief that they will become the adults they want to be.

Arnett (2012) described the 30s and early 40s (up to age 45) as *young adulthood*. He regarded the key characteristic of this stage as *role immersion*, in which marriage or a committed relationship and employment are cemented. It is in young adulthood that role demands are at their highest for most people, with commitments to a partner, children, and work.

It is within the roles and tasks of both emerging and young adulthood that cancer causes significant interruption. For ease of reading, the term *young adult* will be used to describe the individuals who are the focus of this book—those between the ages of 18 and 35.

Concerns of Young Adults With Cancer

Cancer arrests the normal developmental processes of young adults by increasing their dependence on their parents, isolating them from their peers and exposing them to experiences that their peers cannot even imagine, and complicating the establishment of new relationships (Lewis, Jordens, Mooney-Somers, Smith, & Kerridge, 2013). Cancer creates physical burdens, affects future prospects, both in relationships and career opportunities, and brings individuals face to face with their own mortality (Kim & Gillham, 2013). Altered appearance and other body image issues, as well as potential loss of reproductive capacity, are major concerns for young adults with cancer (Zebrack, 2011). However, the cancer experience also has some positive effects, such as strengthened relationships with parents and peers, wisdom and insight beyond that which their peers have experienced at the same age (Lewis et al., 2013), and health competence and future goals (Bellizzi et al., 2012).

It is important to ask young adults what they want or need, as the opinions of their oncology care providers may not correspond with their own needs. For example, in one study, young adults rated the importance of meeting other young cancer survivors higher than their healthcare providers thought they did. These relationships were more important to young adults with cancer than the support they received from their own families and friends (Zebrack, Bleyer, Albritton, Medearis, & Tang, 2006) despite what healthcare providers may think about support from existing relationships.

This study (Zebrack et al., 2006) determined the healthcare needs of young adults and ranked them by importance. Physical needs at the time of diagnosis and during treatment were

1. The presence of a multidisciplinary team that is knowledgeable about young adult needs
2. Treatment decisions that took into account risks to education, fertility, and other quality-of-life issues
3. State-of-the-art treatment protocols and clinical trials specific to young adults
4. Physicians who include cancer in the differential diagnosis when young adults present for care
5. Management of symptoms and side effects of treatment
6. Fertility-preservation services.

Physical needs during survivorship and off-treatment periods were

1. Ongoing surveillance of long-term effects of cancer treatment
2. Transition plans to primary care providers who will adhere to treatment plans
3. Recognition that off-treatment survivorship is a distinct phase of the cancer trajectory
4. Ongoing information for survivors about new treatments and long-term follow-up; tied with the need for evidence-based standards and guidelines for follow-up care.

Another study (Zebrack, Chesler, & Kaplan, 2010) identified the psychosocial needs of young adults in four areas: informational, practical, interpersonal/social, and emotional support. Of note in this study was the need for information that is delivered without condescension and patronization, preparation of the young adults for negative responses from peers and others, and the offer of love and affirmation from healthcare providers.

Quality of Life for Young Adults With Cancer

Although this book does not focus on physical health, it would be remiss to ignore the impact of cancer on quality of life. The latest data from the Adolescent and Young Adult Health Outcomes and Patient Experience (AYA HOPE) study (Smith et al., 2013) show that young adults with cancer have poorer health-related quality of life than their healthy peers with deficits in the areas of physical and emotional roles, physical and social functioning, and fatigue. As would be expected, quality of life is worse during active treatment, for those with current or recent symptoms, and for those without health insurance at any time since they were diagnosed. Those who did not have partners during their cancer experience had the worst mental health.

What This Book Offers

The focus of this book is on the psychosocial needs of young adults with cancer from diagnosis through long-term survivorship and including end-of-life issues. Topics covered include psychosocial needs after diagnosis and during the treatment decision phase; the impact of cancer treatment on dating, relationships, and sexuality; and the potential for impact on fertility. For those who are pregnant at diagnosis, those who become pregnant after cancer, and those who are parenting, the impact of a life-threatening illness poses significant stress. Social relationships with peers, family, and colleagues at work or school also are explored. Recurrence is always possible, and this may mean that the young adult faces the end of life. Distress, an overarching emotion experienced by many, if not all, cancer survivors at some point in the cancer journey, is discussed in its own chapter, as are the supportive care needs of this population.

Although the amount of research in this population is increasing, there remains a paucity of evidence related to effective interventions for young adults with cancer. It is dangerous to assume that what works for older adults can be translated to young adults, especially those on the younger end of the age spectrum. Older adults have greater life experience, are often partnered, have adult children of their own, are facing retirement, and are closer to the end of their lives than the beginning.

References

Arnett, J.J. (2011). Emerging adulthood(s): The cultural psychology of a new life stage. In L.A. Jensen (Ed.), *Bridging cultural and developmental approaches to psychology: New syntheses in theory, research, and policy* (pp. 255–275). New York, NY: Oxford University Press.

Arnett, J.J. (2012). New horizons in research on emerging and young adulthood. In A. Booth, S.L. Brown, N.S. Landale, W.D. Manning, & S.M. McHale (Eds.), *National Symposium on Family Issues: Vol. 2. Early adulthood in a family context* (pp. 231–244). doi:10.1007/978-1-4614-1436-0_15

Bellizzi, K.M., Smith, A., Schmidt, S., Keegan, T.H.M., Zebrack, B., Lynch, C.F., ... Adolescent and Young Adult Health Outcomes and Patient Experience (AYA HOPE) Study Collaborative Group. (2012). Positive and negative psychosocial impact of being diagnosed with cancer as an adolescent or young adult. *Cancer, 118,* 5155–5162. doi:10.1002/cncr.27512

Kim, B., & Gillham, D.M. (2013). The experience of young adult cancer patients described through online narratives. *Cancer Nursing, 36,* 377–384. doi:10.1097/NCC.0b013e318291b4e9

Lewis, P., Jordens, C.F.C., Mooney-Somers, J., Smith, K., & Kerridge, I. (2013). Growing up with cancer: Accommodating the effects of cancer into young people's social lives. *Journal of Pediatric Oncology Nursing, 30,* 311–319. doi:10.1177/1043454213513839

Smith, A.W., Bellizzi, K.M., Keegan, T.H.M., Zebrack, B., Chen, V.W., Neale, A.V., … Lynch, C.F. (2013). Health-related quality of life of adolescent and young adult patients with cancer in the United States: The Adolescent and Young Adult Health Outcomes and Patient Experience study. *Journal of Clinical Oncology, 31,* 2136–2145. doi:10.1200/JCO.2012.47.3173

Zebrack, B., Bleyer, A., Albritton, K., Medearis, S., & Tang, J. (2006). Assessing the health care needs of adolescent and young adult cancer patients and survivors. *Cancer, 107,* 2915–2923. doi:10.1002/cncr.22338

Zebrack, B., Chesler, M.A., & Kaplan, S. (2010). To foster healing among adolescents and young adults with cancer: What helps? What hurts? *Supportive Care in Cancer, 18,* 131–135. doi:10.1007/s00520-009-0719-y

Zebrack, B.J. (2011). Psychological, social, and behavioral issues for young adults with cancer. *Cancer, 117,* 2289–2294. doi:10.1002/cncr.26056

CHAPTER 2
Diagnosis and Treatment Decision Making

Introduction

It is well documented that young adults often experience delayed diagnosis at the start of their cancer journey. The reasons are multifactorial. Diagnostic delay is serious for a number of reasons, including later stage of disease and poorer prognosis because of the delay, as well as loss of trust with the healthcare system. This chapter will describe the factors that influence time to diagnosis and the resulting psychosocial consequences.

Prediagnosis and Diagnosis

Cancer Awareness

Many young adults have not encountered someone with cancer and may not know much about the disease or the signs and symptoms related to it. Their knowledge may be restricted to what they have seen in the media, if they were paying any attention. This lack of awareness may affect their ability to discern the need to report symptoms to a healthcare provider.

Recognition of symptoms and interpretation of them as something serious are factors in delayed diagnosis of cancer. In a review of help-seeking among people with various kinds of cancers, Smith, Pope, and Botha (2005) identified factors that result in a delay in recognizing symptoms suggestive of cancer, which were
- Vague or mild symptoms that were thought to not be serious or need urgent attention
- Absence of pain or lump

- Symptoms that did not persist over time but rather came and went
- Belief that the symptoms would go away
- Lack of awareness of the symptom being related to cancer or risk of cancer.

Cancer awareness in young people is generally low. In a study from the United Kingdom with a sample of 478 adolescents ages 11–17 (Kyle, Forbat, & Hubbard, 2012), 51% of respondents did not know the most common kinds of childhood cancers, and 49% did not know about teenage cancers. The older the adolescents, the more they knew, and if they knew someone with cancer, awareness was greater. In this study, the barriers to seeking medical attention were fearing what might be discovered (72% of participants), feeling embarrassed (56%), being scared (54%), and not feeling confident enough to disclose their symptoms (53%).

Factors Associated With Diagnostic Delay

In addition to a lack of awareness of cancer and its symptoms, other factors contribute to diagnostic delay. These include patient factors and healthcare provider factors.

Gibson et al. (2013) conducted a study to explore the prediagnosis experience of young adults with cancer. The findings of this study are presented in the following paragraphs. An important conclusion of the study was that delays result in a loss of trust in healthcare providers and the system. Patients experienced the loss of time due to delayed diagnosis on multiple levels, including sadness or regret about what has been lost, frustration that the normal ways of being as a young adult are put on hold because of the cancer, and longing for a return to normal life.

Patient Factors

Lack of awareness about cancer, as discussed in the previous section, is an important factor in an individual's delay in help-seeking. In Gibson et al.'s (2013) study, some participants attributed the onset of symptoms to something other than illness. For example, if early symptoms were vague, individuals tended to normalize them or incorporate them into normal life. One young woman in this study had highly suggestive symptoms including rectal bleeding and loss of appetite, but she attributed them to "just who she was." Others minimized symptoms so that their normal life with studying and traveling could continue without interruption. If pain was present, individuals attributed it to accidental trauma and not anything more sinister.

Young adults may seek reassurance from those close to them. In the Gibson et al. (2013) study cited previously, some parents provided reassurance that what they were experiencing was normal or due to some benign reason, but they also encouraged the young adult to seek medical attention.

Friends and other family members may play a similar role. Depending on how they appraise the situation, young adults may either act upon or ignore the encouragement to seek professional help.

Fear is a factor that is cited in the literature as a barrier to seeking care when symptoms are noted (Smith et al., 2005). Fear of embarrassment because the symptoms are related to sexual organs or symptoms may be significant for young adults who are exploring their sexuality. For young men, complaining about a physical symptom may be linked to fears about not being seen as masculine. Furthermore, young adults may fear being perceived as a worrier or a hypochondriac by both healthcare providers and family and friends.

Fear of being diagnosed with cancer also prevents individuals from seeking care. Some people would rather avoid diagnosis because knowing that they have cancer is the worst thing that could happen. This is a form of denial and may lead to late diagnosis of a more advanced cancer. Others may be so fearful of side effects of treatment (e.g., pain, nausea, alterations in sexuality) that they avoid diagnosis. In addition, young adults, because of their need to act independently and their feelings of being invincible, are less likely to seek help when experiencing ill health.

Healthcare Provider Factors

The number of times that someone visits a primary care provider before referral to a specialist is regarded as a measure of the quality of the patient experience (Lyratzopoulos, Neal, Barbiere, Rubin, & Abel, 2012). Young adults ages 16–24 and 25–34 were twice as likely to have three or more visits to their general practitioner before referral than older adults (odds ratio [OR] 2.12, 95% confidence interval [CI] [1.63, 2.75]; and OR 1.82, 95% CI [1.51, 2.20], respectively). In a review of time to diagnosis in young adults, delays occurred in this age group for a variety of reasons, including lack of awareness by general practitioners, the rarity of cancers in this age group, the independence and lack of parental supervision, and lack of knowledge of the healthcare needs of young adults (Lethaby et al., 2013).

Gibson et al. (2013) conducted their study in the United Kingdom, where most of the participants had seen a general practitioner first before eventually being referred to a specialist. However, in North America, many young adults do not have a primary care provider, so access to health care may play a role. Gibson et al. (2013) found that having a general practitioner produced mixed results. For some, it meant a faster referral to specialist care, whereas for others, the referral process was slow and frustrating with multiple visits and a perceived lack of attention to the young adult's complaints. Some of the young adults were seen by another physician in the practice or a locum, and this tended to make them feel as if their complaints were not being taken seriously. Others found that seeing someone who was not familiar with them resulted in more timely referrals. Overall, however, the study participants expressed a sense of frustration and eventual desperation at the time it was taking to get their concerns addressed. And even with timely referrals, there was a lot of "waiting time" for appointments, tests, and test results.

Lyratzopoulos et al. (2012) reported that general practitioners are more likely to refer patients who have symptoms of cancers that are well known or that have well-described characteristics, such as a change in a mole or a new pigmented lesion being suspicious for melanoma. If the patient has a lesion that is easy to palpate (for example, in thyroid or breast cancer), consultation with a specialist is more likely to occur. And when the cancer is known to occur more frequently in an age group, such as testicular cancer in young men, a timely referral is more likely.

Once individuals are referred to a specialist, the process appears to run more smoothly and in a timely manner. Participants in Gibson's study reported a sense of relief once they were seen by an oncologist. The young adult participants felt that their complaints were finally being taken seriously, and further testing and the start of treatment occurred in a timely manner (Gibson et al., 2013).

Results of Diagnostic Delay

Bleyer (2007) reported that survival outcomes for young adults with cancer have not kept pace with those of children and older adults. This is partly attributed to delays in diagnosis, lack of health insurance, and lower participation in clinical trials. Delay in diagnosis results in more advanced cancer when it is eventually diagnosed, as well as diagnoses being made and communicated in the emergency department after a young adult with symptoms of advanced disease seeks care (Fern et al., 2013). Loss of trust in the healthcare system also may occur if the individual had repeated visits to healthcare providers with no response or assurances that symptoms were "normal" or attributed to something benign. Loss of trust may result in suboptimal adherence to treatments or avoidance of treatment altogether because if "the system" got it wrong in the first place, perhaps they are wrong about treatment too.

Implications

Cancer in young adults is rarely preventable, as the risk factors for preventable cancers (tobacco and alcohol use, poor nutrition, sun exposure, lack of physical activity) take years to cause cancer. Cancers linked to environmental factors also occur later in life (Bleyer, 2007). The best that healthcare providers can offer young adults is to be aware that, although it is relatively rare, cancer does occur in those between the ages of 19 and 35 and to not ignore their symptoms when they present for care. While screening and early identification of cancer in this population are important, screening healthy populations is controversial, and no screening tests exist for many of the cancers that are more common in young adults.

Much remains unknown about the diagnostic journey of young adults from the onset of symptoms through the start of treatment and into recovery and survivorship. More research is needed about the prediagnostic stage, as it is with all stages of the cancer journey. Care must be taken to avoid ignoring cardinal symptoms while at the same time avoiding overexposing patients to invasive tests that may put them at risk for immediate or long-term iatrogenic side effects.

Increased awareness about cancers in young adults is needed for both healthcare providers and the lay public. The intent is not to raise panic among healthy adolescents and young adults, but education about symptoms of the most common cancers in this population can be provided in the context of cancer prevention (i.e., avoiding tobacco and limiting alcohol use, reducing sun exposure, preventing sexually transmitted infections, and maintaining a healthy diet and physical activity). Although many healthcare providers are aware of the maxim about hearing hoof beats and assuming it is not a zebra but rather a horse, they also need to avoid delaying diagnosis by assuming that cancer is so rare in young adults that it does not appear on the list of differential diagnoses.

Treatment Decision Making

Treatment decision making can be *physician directed*, in which the decision is made by the physician, who is regarded as the expert; *shared*, with the patient and family actively participating in the process; or *patient driven* (the least common form), in which the patient makes a treatment decision independently. It has become the norm for patients to be involved in treatment decision making, and many patients expect to be part of the process. Patients who are part of the decision-making process are more satisfied with their care and experience less regret about the decision. Very little research exists on treatment decision making in young adults with cancer; however, it is generally accepted that younger patients (younger than age 60) want more involvement in treatment decisions than older adults. A great deal of difference exists between young adults and those younger than 60; the studies cited in this chapter all include participants younger than age 35.

Shared Decision Making

Shared decision making is described as a collaborative process that is interactive and characterized by the healthcare provider asking for and acknowledging the patient's preference for participation in the process; giving the patient choices about how the process of making a treatment decision will be made; and mutual respect for the choices that are made (Charles, Gafni, & Whelan, 1997). The guiding principle for this process is the patient's right to self-determination, as well as the expectation that the patient will adhere to the treatment if he or she is involved in the choice (Stalmeier, 2011).

In a national survey in England evaluating the experience of decision-making involvement of more than 41,000 people with cancer, 72% reported positive experiences (El Turabi, Abel, Roland, & Lyratzopoulos, 2013). However, young adult patients reported significantly more negative experiences than adults older than age 65. The researchers concluded that younger patients may have greater expectations for their involvement and therefore are less satisfied if those expectations are not met. Younger patients also may have a greater need for autonomy because they have recently attained independence because of their age. The researchers questioned whether younger patients may be treated differently; however, how their treatment may be different was not explored. In this study, those diagnosed with testicular cancer and melanoma had a more positive experience with decision making. It was postulated that this might be because these are cancers with obvious symptoms and are diagnosed promptly with a generally good prognosis.

In a national survey in the United States (N = 488), shared decision making was associated with satisfaction with the treatment decision, particularly in the areas of patient understanding, solicitation of patient preferences for treatment, and weighing treatment options thoroughly (Glass et al., 2012). This speaks to the quality of the interaction with the healthcare provider, a topic that will be discussed later in this chapter.

Moreau et al. (2012) conducted a study in which scenarios were presented to focus groups of participants, including a group of students. One of the scenarios involved people with cancer. Although these were hypothetical situations, participants saw decision making about treatment as something that should be shared with the physician. They also thought that patients should assess the physician, ask for a second opinion, and consider alternatives to the proposed treatment. A number of other factors were involved in decision making for these participants, including trust, being able to take the time to think, and the quality of the physician's nonverbal communication. Obstacles to shared decision making included serious or emergent health conditions, perception that the physician has inadequate knowledge, fear of the information that might be provided to the patients, and difficulty in asserting oneself and making requests of the physician. While this study has limited application because of the hypothetical nature of the clinical scenarios presented, the recognition that shared decision making may not be possible in emergent or serious conditions has implications for shared decision making in cancer.

In another study that included a small number of young adults (Keating et al., 2010), patients controlled decision making mostly when the benefits of treatment were uncertain. The highest rates of physician control were seen when there was no evidence to support treatment, and the highest rate of shared decision making occurred when there was evidence for treatment. The latter finding suggests that when there is evidence for treatment, physicians may be more likely to share knowledge with the patient, in contrast to situations where evidence is lacking and the physician takes control to prevent unnecessary treatment.

Decision Making in Uncertain Situations

Breast cancer is one situation where there is some choice of treatment (e.g., mastectomy versus lumpectomy and radiation, immediate versus delayed reconstruction) and, for young women, where decisions about fertility preservation need to be made. It also is an area where research specific to younger patients is available. It often is assumed that younger women will take an active role in decision making when diagnosed with breast cancer. In a study from France about decisions to receive chemotherapy and adjuvant endocrine therapy, 20.7% of the women in the study preferred to play a passive role in the decision about further treatment (Seror et al., 2013). This was associated with playing a passive role about surgery as the initial treatment. Women who played a passive role tended to have lower quality of life. Single women in this study preferred a more active role in decision making.

Treatment of breast cancer has the potential to affect future fertility, an area where patient decision making takes on significant importance. A full discussion about fertility can be found in Chapter 6. The focus in the following paragraphs is on the process of decision making relative to fertility concerns.

Women often are more concerned about surviving the cancer than preserving fertility. In a qualitative study of young women with breast cancer, just 12% of young breast cancer survivors reported that fertility was a consideration in the decision they made about treatment (Gorman, Usita, Madlensky, & Pierce, 2011). The dominant concern for many women with breast cancer is the risk of recurrence.

In the same study by Gorman et al. (2011), participants reported that they perceived having little choice in which treatments they had, relying heavily on their oncologists and wanting aggressive treatment to reduce the chance of recurrence. The concept of fertility was dependent on life circumstances for many of the women. Those who expected to have children in the future or who were trying to conceive at the time of the breast cancer diagnosis were more likely to consider the impact of treatment on fertility when making a treatment decision. Some of the women in this study regretted that fertility preservation was not discussed at the time of diagnosis because in retrospect they would have made different treatment decisions had they been more fully informed.

Hershberger, Finnegan, Pierce, and Scoccia (2013) identified clinician behaviors that were helpful or not helpful for women as part of the decision-making process about fertility and treatment. Active listening, open and honest communication perceived by the woman as nonjudgmental, and a respectful environment were factors that enhanced the discussion about fertility issues. Negative factors included clinicians who appeared to be judgmental or insensitive, as well as clinicians who appeared to have an agenda, for example, those who tried to pressure women into preserving fertility or those who advised against it.

Healthcare Providers and Decision Making

In reality, physicians set the agenda for treatment decision making. They are the guardians of the information from pathology reports and investigations and possess privileged knowledge about treatment options. It has traditionally been the sole responsibility of the physician to convey a diagnosis; however, this has changed with the introduction of advanced practice nurses, physician assistants, and other providers who may do this in some jurisdictions. Little information exists about the role of healthcare providers other than physicians in disclosing a cancer diagnosis to a person who then becomes a patient.

It might be easier for healthcare providers to communicate with their patients when there is certainty about the disease and its prognosis and the treatment is clear with little or no choice. When uncertainty exists, patients may be dissatisfied with the decision-making process and more anxious. However, patients who are involved in treatment decision making are less dissatisfied than those who are not involved and who are treated by physicians with a paternalistic attitude (Politi, Clark, Ombao, Dizon, & Elwyn, 2011).

In a study of Australian oncologists (Shepherd, Butow, & Tattersall, 2011), physicians' willingness to participate in shared decision making was dependent on cancer specialty (specific cancers treated) and discipline (medical oncologist vs. radiation oncologist vs. surgeon). The physicians in this study described the following five features of the cancer that influence how information is shared and decisions about treatment are made.

- The context of the decision: Some decisions are seen as clear-cut, where there is only one treatment; in these cases, patients are less likely to be involved. Other decisions are more ambiguous, and patients are more likely to be involved in these instances.
- Existence of treatment options: In these cases, patients usually are involved in making the decision. Where protocols or guidelines are available, patient

involvement is less likely to occur. In emergent situations, such as acute leukemia, physicians are not likely to engage patients in a discussion, as this is seen as a waste of time and a potential threat to the patient's life.

- Impact of treatment on the patient: The greater the impact of treatment on the patient's lifestyle and self-image, the more likely the physician would be to involve the patient. Treatment for breast cancer was cited as an example of where treatment could alter body image and sexuality, and physicians did not want to impose their values and judgment on the patient.
- Disease culture: Patients with cancers that have active advocacy groups (e.g., breast cancer) are seen to be more interested in participating in shared decision making, whereas patients with less well-known cancers (e.g., leukemia) are seen as not knowing enough to be actively involved in decision making or as having unrealistic expectations of treatment.
- Stage of disease: Physicians are more likely to involve patients in treatment decision making when the prognosis is good or when the cancer has advanced and no more evidence-based treatments are available.

How to Help the Young Adult With Cancer

Patient-centered communication is recognized as an important aspect of care and shared decision making and is increasingly being incorporated into educational programs for healthcare providers. Not all healthcare providers are expert communicators. Although younger providers have received training in communication to enhance interactions with patients, older healthcare providers often have not and may have a style that is paternalistic or at least not patient-centered.

The central tenet of patient-centered communication is a focus on patients and their values and the context of their lives. A recent Cochrane review on the topic (Dwamena et al., 2012) suggested that training programs of less than 10 hours are effective in teaching healthcare providers new communication skills; however, the subsequent effect on patients is limited. Health information technology (HIT) in the form of decision aids and disease management systems also has been shown to improve outcomes for patients, particularly in the areas of enhanced provider-patient relationships and care management (Finkelstein et al., 2012). This review highlighted that using HIT improves outcomes for people with cancer by increasing the responsiveness to individuals' preferences and needs. Given that most young adults today are technology natives, using HIT with this population may be very effective.

Evidence of the effectiveness of HIT was shown in a study of a psychoeducational video game in adolescents and young adults with cancer (Beale, Kato, Marin-Bowling, Guthrie, & Cole, 2007). The game, called Re-Mission, features an avatar that travels through the bodies of 19 different patients being treated for the seven most common cancers in young people. The avatar has a companion robot that provides information, encouragement, and warnings as the avatar destroys cancer cells, bacteria, and viruses using common treatments such as radiation and chemotherapy. Players must also use prompts that encourage positive behaviors such as medication adherence and other self-care activities. The game, along with a second version called Re-Mission 2, is available at www.re-mission.net. The study showed that knowledge about cancer and its treatments was significantly improved in the group that used the video game compared to the control group.

However, barriers to the use of HIT exist. These include problems accessing the technology, such as an unappealing interface or usability problems, as well as sociodemographic factors, such as low income and cognitive impairment. The skill of healthcare providers in working with HIT is of concern, as low computer literacy and lack of formal training may prevent providers from recommending programs to patients. Physicians have also raised concerns about funding, workload, and workflow demands as barriers to the use of HIT (Finkelstein et al., 2012).

Decision aids, including decision boards, computer-based interventions, audio recordings, and pamphlets, are well established in clinical practice for a number of screening tests and other procedures. In their review, Spiegle et al. (2013) concluded that simpler tools (e.g., prompt lists) may be as effective as more involved decision aids. Use of a decision aid may increase knowledge and patient satisfaction but does not reduce anxiety or decisional conflict.

An updated Cochrane review (Stacey et al., 2014) concluded that decision aids are useful when treatment options exist for a particular condition, when there is no clear outcome advantage of one option over another, and when there are harms and benefits associated with the treatments that individuals may value differently. This review found that when decision aids are used to help patients make treatment decisions, knowledge is improved, patients have more accurate expectations of potential benefits and harms, they make choices that are more reflective of their values, and they are more active participants in decision making.

The Ottawa Hospital Research Institute has an alphabetical list of patient decision aids, including many for cancer. The institute reviewed the decision aids according to the International Patient Decision Aid Standards. This list, including links to specific decision aids, is available at https://decisionaid.ohri.ca/AZlist.html.

Conclusion

The diagnosis of cancer in young adults is always a life-altering event, and for some, it will be a life-threatening one. There is no preparation for the receipt of a cancer diagnosis, and the resultant upheaval in the lives of young adults can have far-reaching consequences. There is an expectation today that patients will be involved in making decisions about their treatment, and this chapter has focused on the experience of patients regarding this process and strategies to help young adults negotiate their way through the process.

References

Beale, I.L., Kato, P.M., Marin-Bowling, V.M., Guthrie, N., & Cole, S.W. (2007). Improvement in cancer-related knowledge following use of a psychoeducational video game for adolescents and young adults with cancer. *Journal of Adolescent Health, 41,* 263–270. doi:10.1016/j.jadohealth.2007.04.006

Bleyer, A. (2007). Young adult oncology: The patients and their survival challenges. *CA: A Cancer Journal for Clinicians, 57,* 242–255. doi:10.3322/canjclin.57.4.242

Charles, C., Gafni, A., & Whelan, T. (1997). Shared decision-making in the medical encounter: What does it mean? (or it takes at least two to tango). *Social Science and Medicine, 44,* 681–692. doi:10.1016/S0277-9536(96)00221-3

Dwamena, F., Holmes-Rovner, M., Gaulden, C.M., Jorgenson, S., Sadigh, G., Sikorskii, A., ... Beasley, M. (2012). Interventions for providers to promote a patient-centred approach in clinical consultations. *Cochrane Database of Systematic Reviews, 2012*(12). doi:10.1002/14651858.CD003267.pub2

El Turabi, A., Abel, G.A., Roland, M., & Lyratzopoulos, G. (2013). Variation in reported experience of involvement in cancer treatment decision making: Evidence from the National Cancer Patient Experience Survey. *British Journal of Cancer, 109,* 780–787. doi:10.1038/bjc.2013.316

Fern, L.A., Birch, R., Whelan, J., Cooke, M., Sutton, S., Neal, R.D., ... Gibson, F. (2013). Why can't we improve the timeliness of cancer diagnosis in children, teenagers, and young adults? *BMJ, 347,* f6493. doi:10.1136/bmj.f6493

Finkelstein, J., Knight, A., Marinopoulos, S., Gibbons, M.C., Berger, Z., Aboumatar, H., ... Bass, E.B. (2012). *Enabling patient-centered care through health information technology* (Evidence Report/Technology Assessment No. 206, AHRQ Publication No. 12-E005-EF). Rockville, MD: Agency for Healthcare Research and Quality.

Gibson, F., Pearce, S., Eden, T., Glaser, A., Hooker, L., Whelan, J., & Kelly, D. (2013). Young people describe their prediagnosis cancer experience. *Psycho-Oncology, 22,* 2585–2592. doi:10.1002/pon.3325

Glass, K.E., Wills, C.E., Holloman, C., Olson, J., Hechmer, C., Miller, C.K., & Duchemin, A.-M. (2012). Shared decision making and other variables as correlates of satisfaction with health care decisions in a United States national survey. *Patient Education and Counseling, 88,* 100–105. doi:10.1016/j.pec.2012.02.010

Gorman, J.R., Usita, P.M., Madlensky, L., & Pierce, J.P. (2011). Young breast cancer survivors: Their perspectives on treatment decisions and fertility concerns. *Cancer Nursing, 34,* 32–40. doi:10.1097/NCC.0b013e3181e4528d

Hershberger, P.E., Finnegan, L., Pierce, P.F., & Scoccia, B. (2013). The decision-making process of young adult women with cancer who considered fertility cryopreservation. *Journal of Obstetric, Gynecologic, and Neonatal Nursing, 42,* 59–69. doi:10.1111/j.1552-6909.2012.01426.x

Keating, N.L., Landrum, M.B., Arora, N.K., Malin, J.L., Ganz, P.A., van Ryn, M., & Weeks, J.C. (2010). Cancer patients' roles in treatment decisions: Do characteristics of the decision influence roles? *Journal of Clinical Oncology, 28,* 4364–4370. doi:10.1200/JCO.2009.26.8870

Kyle, R.G., Forbat, L., & Hubbard, G. (2012). Cancer awareness among adolescents in Britain: A cross-sectional study. *BMC Public Health, 12,* 580. doi:10.1186/1471-2458-12-580

Lethaby, C.D., Picton, S., Kinsey, S.E., Phillips, R., van Laar, M., & Feltbower, R.G. (2013). A systematic review of time to diagnosis in children and young adults with cancer. *Archives of Disease in Childhood, 98,* 349–355. doi:10.1136/archdischild-2012-303034

Lyratzopoulos, G., Neal, R.D., Barbiere, J.M., Rubin, G.P., & Abel, G.A. (2012). Variation in number of general practitioner consultations before hospital referral for cancer: Findings from the 2010 National Cancer Patient Experience Survey in England. *Lancet Oncology, 13,* 353–365. doi:10.1016/S1470-2045(12)70041-4

Moreau, A., Carol, L., Dedianne, M.C., Dupraz, C., Perdrix, C., Lainé, X., & Souweine, G. (2012). What perceptions do patients have of decision making (DM)? Toward an integrative patient-centered care model. A qualitative study using focus-group interviews. *Patient Education and Counseling, 87,* 206–211. doi:10.1016/j.pec.2011.08.010

Politi, M.C., Clark, M.A., Ombao, H., Dizon, D., & Elwyn, G. (2011). Communicating uncertainty can lead to less decision satisfaction: A necessary cost of involving patients in shared decision making? *Health Expectations, 14,* 84–91. doi:10.1111/j.1369-7625.2010.00626.x

Seror, V., Cortaredona, S., Bouhnik, A.-D., Meresse, M., Cluze, C., Viens, P., ... Peretti-Watel, P. (2013). Young breast cancer patients' involvement in treatment decisions: The major role played by decision-making about surgery. *Psycho-Oncology, 22,* 2546–2556. doi:10.1002/pon.3316

Shepherd, H.L., Butow, P.N., & Tattersall, M.H.N. (2011). Factors which motivate cancer doctors to involve their patients in reaching treatment decisions. *Patient Education and Counseling, 84,* 229–235. doi:10.1016/j.pec.2010.10.018

Smith, L.K., Pope, C., & Botha, J.L. (2005). Patients' help-seeking experiences and delay in cancer presentation: A qualitative synthesis. *Lancet, 366,* 825–831. doi:10.1016/S0140-6736(05)67030-4

Spiegle, G., Al-Sukhni, E., Schmocker, S., Gagliardi, A.R., Victor, J.C., Baxter, N.N., & Kennedy, E.D. (2013). Patient decision aids for cancer treatment: Are there any alternatives? *Cancer, 119,* 189–200. doi:10.1002/cncr.27641

Stacey, D., Légaré, F., Col, N.F., Bennett, C.L., Barry, M.J., Eden, K.B., ... Wu, J.H.C. (2014). Decision aids for people facing health treatment or screening decisions. *Cochrane Database of Systematic Reviews, 2014*(1). doi:10.1002/14651858.CD001431.pub4

Stalmeier, P.F.M. (2011). Adherence and decision aids: A model and a narrative review. *Medical Decision Making, 31,* 121–129. doi:10.1177/0272989X10370487

CHAPTER 3
Treatment

Introduction

Young adults with cancer are frequently described as being "lost in transition" because they fall between the disciplines of pediatric and adult oncology. Nowhere is this more apparent than during active treatment. Discrepancies exist between where these young people are treated—pediatric inpatient units versus adult inpatient units or outpatient facilities—as well as by whom. Some debate also exists about whether to treat young adults by following pediatric or adult protocols and guidelines.

The psychosocial needs of this population are complex. These needs may be heightened during the active treatment phase when the individuals are experiencing the acute side effects of treatment. The loss of independence and connection with their peer group is especially concerning during periods of inpatient care.

This chapter will describe the challenges of providing treatment to young adults and the experiences of young adults with hospital admission. The voices of their parents will be included, as well as some creative interventions to make this challenging time better for all concerned.

Treatment-Related Issues

The National Comprehensive Cancer Network® (2014) guidelines identify the following issues related to treatment of adolescents and young adults.

- Dose schedules: Young adults are able to tolerate more intensive treatment doses than older adults, and more intensive therapy is associated with improved outcomes.
- Toxicities: Screening for cardiac, renal, and neurologic toxicity is very important.

- Fertility: Fertility preservation should be an essential part of the management of young adults.
- Psychosocial and behavioral considerations: Healthcare providers need to recognize, assess for, and treat psychosocial and behavioral issues.

The guidelines also address psychosocial issues affecting young adults with cancer undergoing treatment with suggestions for potential interventions. These include assessment of the following factors.

- Individual: Cognitive function, emotional distress, living status, treatment adherence, work/school, substance use, sexual concerns (including risky behavior), nutrition, exercise, spiritual issues
- Relationships: Family, peers, communication, decision making, information sharing
- Socioeconomic: Insurance, child care, transportation, complementary and alternative medicine use

The Livestrong Young Adult Alliance (sponsored by the Livestrong Foundation and the National Cancer Institute) recommended that all healthcare providers who care for young adults with cancer should be educated in three areas: medical knowledge specific to young adults, care delivery that is specific to young adults and not associated with pediatric or older adult care, and competency in providing young adult–specific practical knowledge (Hayes-Lattin, Mathews-Bradshaw, & Siegel, 2010). This position statement suggested multiple avenues for educating healthcare personnel, including seminars at oncology conferences, specific courses in undergraduate and graduate curricula, postgraduate courses and fellowships, and continuing education opportunities.

Where Should Young Adults With Cancer Be Treated?

Where to treat young adults with cancer is an ongoing conundrum. Should they be treated in pediatric clinics and units, where many of the other patients will be of preschool age? Or should they be admitted to adult inpatient units and clinics, where the average patient is older than 60? The treatment of older adults in the United States often occurs in community oncology clinics rather than cancer centers. It has been suggested that multidisciplinary care provided in academic treatment centers with access to a variety of specialists and supportive care services may be more appropriate for young adults (Ferrari et al., 2010).

Young adults with cancer are not going to feel comfortable in either of these traditional locations. The culture of the inpatient unit or clinic is also a challenge. In pediatric clinics, patients' parents are intimately involved in decision making and in monitoring disease progression or recovery. Patient resources are focused on young children, with child-life specialists, teachers, and social workers as part of the team. The physical space in a pediatric unit usually has cartoon characters on the walls and clowns and other entertainers as distractions in waiting rooms or visiting patients in their rooms. Adult inpatient and clinic spaces tend to be utilitarian and more somber (Ferrari et al., 2010). It is unusual to see young children in adult units; however, young adults with cancer may have young children who will visit or accompany them, and the presence of young children or babies may be disconcerting for other patients and staff.

Provider expertise is another factor to consider. Pediatric oncologists, nurses, and allied healthcare providers may not be trained in the specific age-related and developmental-stage needs of young adults. The sharing of health information and treatment decision making with pediatric patients usually involves the parent or parents of the child; however, young adults may not want their parents involved in these areas at all. Conversely, in adult units, autonomy is assumed, but some young adults may not want complete independence when making important decisions. Depending on patients' maturity level and cognitive abilities, the care of adolescents and young adults may require more parental involvement than adult oncology providers are accustomed to (Ferrari et al., 2010).

In addition, adult oncologists may not have the expertise to deal with the pediatric treatment protocols that are recommended for young adults and may be less likely to treat this population as aggressively as their pediatric colleagues are trained to do (Albritton & Bleyer, 2003).

Transitioning Care

The journey for all individuals with cancer comprises multiple transitions from diagnosis to active treatment, then to the end of treatment, and finally to long-term follow-up and survivorship care (Nathan, Hayes-Lattin, Sisler, & Hudson, 2011). However, additional challenges for young adults with cancer arise with each of these transitions because of the normal developmental tasks and required milestone achievements associated with their stage of life. The most significant transition for young adults with cancer may be the move from pediatric or young adult care to adult services for long-term follow-up.

McInally (2013) suggested that transitioning young adults into adult care requires specific and detailed care pathways and the services of healthcare providers who are educated and have a passion for this work. She further suggested that communication among healthcare providers needs to be consistent and should start ahead of the actual transition. Care must be family centered and not defined only by age but rather according to the needs of individual patients.

Experiences of Young Adults and Their Parents

Cancer is an unexpected intruder in the lives of young adults. Once the shock of diagnosis has been overcome, the usually rapid initiation of treatment poses yet another set of challenges. The treatment experience of young adults with cancer has been summed up in one word: isolation. Treatment involves isolation from their peers and community, isolation from others with the same disease in treatment at the same time because of the rarity of cancer in this population, and isolation from the treatment team, who may not be experienced in caring for this population and may not be comfortable communicating with them. Young adults also are isolated from research and expertise because of the small number of patients in this age group, and experience caring for them may be limited by location of the treatment center (Thomas, Seymour, O'Brien, Sawyer, & Ashley, 2006).

Thompson, Palmer, and Dyson (2009) described concerns of young adults in three broad categories: information processing and communication, the treatment process, and post-treatment care and survivorship. They identified issues in each of these categories as follows.

- Information processing and communication
  - Healthcare providers did not deliver information about diagnosis and treatment in a manner that was understood by young adults.
  - Healthcare providers did not deliver important information about fertility preservation in a timely manner.
- The treatment process
  - The healthcare team did not provide skilled and timely interventions for physical and psychological challenges such as sexuality and body image.
- Post-treatment care and survivorship
  - Young adults expressed significant concerns about ending treatment and leaving the safety of the acute setting.
  - Young adults reported fears of recurrence and uncertainty about the future.

In a large study of almost 300 young adult survivors (Zebrack et al., 2014), participants described dissatisfaction with the location of their treatment—adult or pediatric units—and confusion with coordination of care. This was echoed in a study from the United Kingdom (Grinyer, 2009) in which young adults reported that the location of care was important and that it affected their morale, adherence, and potentially their treatment outcomes. This study compared the attitudes of young adults with those of their parents and raised some interesting issues related to medical information and who "owned" this information. For parents, the pressing priority was the survival of their child, and location of treatment was of little importance. Some parents in this study requested that a poor prognosis not be disclosed to their young adult child in case the individual then refused treatment; the parents wanted their young adult child to have any chance of survival, even if this meant aggressive and ultimately futile treatment. The young adults, however, wanted to maintain their independence and to own their medical information and treatment decision-making role.

Financial Challenges

Financial issues, specifically lack of health insurance, can be a significant barrier and stressor for young adults with cancer. While individuals younger than 18 are eligible for Medicaid coverage (McInally, 2013), young adults who are older than that may experience barriers to access because of their inability to pay for medical care. In a study of 465 young adults with cancer, Keegan et al. (2014) found that those without insurance were less likely to see a healthcare provider. Forty-four percent did not seek medical care because it was either too expensive or they did not have insurance. Many young adults who are treated in hospital-based cancer centers will receive care regardless of their ability to pay because their care is supported by financial assistance through charity or nonprofit organizations.

The Patient Protection and Affordable Care Act of 2010 is anticipated to be beneficial for young adults with cancer. First, it allows young adults up to age 26 to remain on their parents' insurance plan and does not permit withdrawal of coverage (Moy et al., 2011). Even if young adults have health insurance, other financial issues may negatively affect their access to care. These include co-payments, deductibles, out-of-pocket expenses for treatment-related items, and costs for transportation and child care, as well as lost wages and student loan obligations.

How to Help the Young Adult With Cancer

Navigating Treatment and Survivorship

Given that young adults struggle with the issues described previously, how best can healthcare professionals help them to navigate the treatment period and subsequent transition to survivorship care? Thompson et al. (2009) suggested the following.

- Continuous contact with the treating oncologist should occur for at least a year after the end of treatment. This will reduce any feelings of abandonment and mitigate the need for repeating their cancer history to new providers.

- A survivorship care plan should be provided, with contribution from the young adults in its creation. This is theorized to increase confidence in self-management.
- The healthcare team should provide young adults assistance with reintegration into their community, including educational and vocational support and psychosocial support as needed.
- Clinicians should regularly assess not only the physical effects of treatment but also psychosocial needs and quality of life.
- Supportive care should be offered on a regular basis and delivered by providers who are experts in the care of young adults to enable individuals to return to a new normal life after the upheaval of cancer diagnosis and treatment.
- Surveillance for late effects of cancer should be clearly explained to young adult survivors so that they can be active participants in their own care. The need for specialist care may occur years from initial treatment, and new symptoms should be dealt with promptly.
- Opportunities for peer support should be encouraged during active treatment, when possible, and in the survivorship phase.
- Return to school or work should be facilitated with teachers, professors, and employers wherever possible. This may involve education for classmates and coworkers, but only with the consent of the survivor.

The question of where young adults should be treated involves economic and logistical challenges. The United Kingdom led the world in recognizing the unique needs of this population with the establishment of the Teenage Cancer Trust. Several adolescent and young adult units have been established in the United Kingdom; however, similar initiatives in the United States have been limited.

To date, only the Seattle Children's Hospital has established an inpatient unit that caters to young adults. The rooms have patient-controlled mood lighting and are designed to protect privacy. A couch is available for parents to sleep on, but a privacy curtain separates the patient's bed from this area. Each room also has two televisions so that patients and their parents or other visitors can watch different programs at the same time, and Internet access is available. Visiting hours end at midnight to accommodate friends who want to visit late into the night. Each room also has a small refrigerator and a private shower (Seattle Children's Hospital, n.d.).

Other hospitals have made efforts to be more inclusive of the needs of young adults, including setting up special lounges and recreation areas for adolescents and young adults (MD Anderson Cancer Center in Houston, Texas), creating a Teen Room and Teen Nights (Hyundai Cancer Institute at the Children's Hospital of Orange County, California), and establishing consultation services or clinics at a number of other cancer centers and hospitals.

Olsen and Harder (2011) described the efforts that nurses in the youth unit at a university hospital in Denmark made to create a therapeutic environment for their patients. The nursing staff's aim was to strengthen the social networks of young adult patients during their hospitalization so that they continued to grow and develop despite their illness. The nurses did this by a process they called *bridging*. Bridging encompassed linking and moving across or over obstacles in an effort to facilitate the social networks in which growth occurs. Nursing strategies that encouraged this included tuning in, framing the situation, navigating toward the goal, and connecting people (see Figure 3-1).

Tuning in refers to creating a good rapport, establishing confidentiality, and using open communication in order to be invited into the private world of young adult patients. Three processes are involved in tuning in: (a) getting on the same wavelength, (b) embracing a different social convention, and (c) facing a broader spectrum.

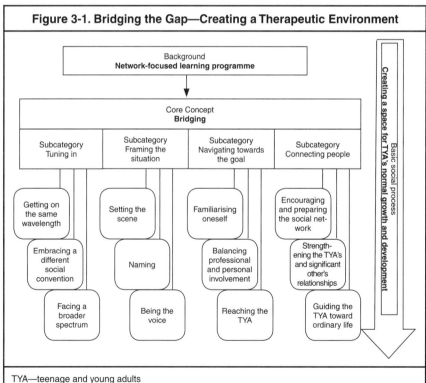

Figure 3-1. Bridging the Gap—Creating a Therapeutic Environment

TYA—teenage and young adults

Note. From "Caring for Teenagers and Young Adults With Cancer: A Grounded Theory Study of Network-Focused Nursing," by P.R. Olsen and I. Harder, 2011, *European Journal of Oncology Nursing, 15,* p. 155. doi:10.1016/j.ejon.2010.07.01. Copyright 2011 by Elsevier. Reprinted with permission.

- In order to *get on the same wavelength*, nurses used strategies such as creating a youthful environment, asking about friends and leisure time activities, and using humor and jokes. The nurses were at times challenged by the patients' use of television, computers, and cell phones, but with time, they realized that the patients could multitask and did not have to make eye contact to pay attention. Older nurses found themselves in the role of mother figure, which at times was a barrier, while younger nurses were considered as friends by the patients. The nurses found that conversations became deeper and more intimate late at night, and they felt like they were substitute friends at these times.
- *Embracing a different social convention* refers to the way that the nurses let go of their usual communication styles and interactions and were freer and less formal with these younger patients. The nurses found that the constant presence of family was sometimes helpful but also led to a feeling of being watched constantly.
- *Facing a broader spectrum* relates to the contact with family members. For the nurses, this occasionally made them feel as though they were caring for more than one patient. This also allowed for more questions and conversations, which took more of the nurses' time, so they had to plan their care accordingly.

Framing the situation refers to being clear in communication with patients and being truthful and open about the challenges that lay ahead for the young adult and the family. This involves three processes: (a) setting the scene, (b) naming, and (c) being the voice.

- *Setting the scene* describes the way that nurses expressed their personal ideas and values. This included respect for the autonomy of their young patients and advocating on their behalf.
- *Naming* refers to the way that the nurses talked about topics that were taboo and also in the consistency with which all the nurses talked about the illness with the patients and families so that everyone heard the same information.
- *Being the voice* refers to nurses' asking patients about what to include in meeting their needs regarding care and progress.

Navigating toward the goal refers to nurses moving outside of their traditional roles in promoting the social network and being involved in more private aspects of their patients' lives. At the same time, they had to balance this with the risk of becoming too close to the patient and family. This was accomplished by the following three processes: (a) familiarizing oneself, (b) balancing professional and personal involvement, and (c) reaching the teenager and young adult.

- *Familiarizing oneself* with the patient and family required observation of the family dynamics and roles during the early days of the patient's admission. This allowed for mutual understanding and the development of trust. The end goal of this was to create the most supportive conditions for young adults during their time in the hospital.

- *Balancing professional and personal involvement* was a challenging task, especially for younger nurses who risked losing their objectivity if they too closely identified as a friend to the patient and jeopardized their role as a nurse. Over time the nurses felt that they were bonded to the patient and family, and this connection endured even past the treatment period and the death of some patients.
- *Reaching the teenager and young adult* was difficult for the nurses, especially when parents overstepped their boundaries and tried to take control from their child. This resulted in the patients becoming passive, which challenged the nurses who continued to treat the young adults with respect and autonomously.

The final category in this description is that of **connecting people**. The nurses tried to do this by means of a network meeting where family and friends could hear what the young adult needed and identify ways of meeting these needs. The processes involved in this were (a) encouraging and preparing the social network, (b) strengthening relationships with others, and (c) guiding the teenager or young adult toward ordinary life.

- *Encouraging and preparing the social network* was accomplished by telling members of a patient's social networks what they could do to help the patient and his or her family. This included giving them small tasks to do and emphasizing how important this support was to the patient and family.
- *Strengthening relationships with others* refers to the efforts the nurses made to persuade the patients to participate in the regular aspects of their life and how to deal with problems related to the cancer and its treatment. The nurses also found themselves supporting the families and helping them to see how they were helping the patients.
- *Guiding the teenager or young adult toward ordinary life* was seen as essential in helping patients make plans for the future when they tended to withdraw and isolate themselves.

Although this may appear to be an intensive and perhaps extraordinary effort, many important lessons and exemplars from this paper can guide the nursing care of young adult patients. Key issues include building trust with patients and their families, encouraging a strong support network for patients and families, advocating for patients' autonomy, and helping patients plan for their future. These are all doable and do not require financial resources outside of time and effort.

The Ideal Young Adult Unit

What constitutes an ideal unit for young adults with cancer? Certainly the physical environment would be an important aspect of inpatient care. Suggestions include private rooms and bathrooms, wireless Internet, access to fresh food and snacks when desired, the ability to have friends visit beyond visiting hours, a separate lounge area where patients can meet outside of their rooms, recreational space and activities (e.g., movie nights, games), and access to a gym for regular exercise. However, these are merely window dressing if the culture of the unit does not take into account the unique needs and developmental milestones of this population.

The attitudes of staff in any unit, inpatient or outpatient, need to be distinctly different when caring for young adults as compared to older adults or children. Staff need to have a very real understanding of the developmental stage of emerging and young adults and tailor their care and education accordingly. Young adults are risk takers by nature, although variation exists between those on the younger end of the spectrum as compared to those in their 30s. Adherence to treatment protocols, especially those that are patient controlled such as oral anticancer agents, may be tenuous. Healthcare providers should explore patients' reasons for nonadherence rather than criticizing or judging.

An attitude of "starting from yes" can be a valuable asset when working with young adult patients. Instead of assuming that something cannot be done (most often because it has never been tried before), starting from considering or acquiescing to a request can close the gap between what the young adult patient wants and what is actually possible. An example of this is day or night passes so that the patient can go to a concert or party. As long as leaving the unit does not pose a threat to the patient's life, the healthcare team can make adjustments to dosing or IV treatments with a little effort. Patients may have to sign a contract that they will not do anything to jeopardize their health (such as drinking alcohol or taking recreational drugs). Patients have to be medically stable to go out on passes and understand they are responsible for their own health while they are out of the hospital. They need to have a fully charged cell phone so they can call for help if necessary and need to know whom to call if they encounter any difficulties or do not feel well while away.

It is vital that young adult patients are allies and active participants in their own care. When much of their control over their lives has been lost because of cancer, it is even more important to give them control over other aspects of their life. For example, when to eat and what to eat may seem unimportant, but if this is the only choice in a young person's life, it is a very important choice, and care should be taken to ensure that this choice is provided.

The efforts of the nurses from Denmark (Olsen & Harder, 2011) and their creation of a culture of acceptance and appropriate care for young adults suggest the magnitude of the cultural shift that is necessary to provide meaningful care to this population. The results might be well worth the effort for both staff and patients.

Conclusion

The question of where to treat young adults with cancer is not a philosophical one; the location and culture of the treatment unit can have important psychosocial ramifications for the young adults and their family members. It is also one influenced by economics and the larger healthcare system. Not every treatment center or hospital has the ability to create special spaces for young adults. If young adults live close to an academic center, they may receive more appropriate care there, where the treatment teams may have more experience in treating young adults and patients may have the opportunity to meet others of their age with cancer.

References

Albritton, K., & Bleyer, W.A. (2003). The management of cancer in the older adolescent. *European Journal of Cancer, 39*, 2584–2599. doi:10.1016/j.ejca.2003.09.013

Ferrari, A., Thomas, D., Franklin, A.R.K., Hayes-Lattin, B.M., Mascarin, M., van der Graaf, W., & Albritton, K.H. (2010). Starting an adolescent and young adult program: Some success stories and some obstacles to overcome. *Journal of Clinical Oncology, 28*, 4850–4857. doi:10.1200/JCO.2009.23.8097

Grinyer, A. (2009). Contrasting parental perspectives with those of teenagers and young adults with cancer: Comparing the findings from two qualitative studies. *European Journal of Oncology Nursing, 13*, 200–206. doi:10.1016/j.ejon.2009.04.002

Hayes-Lattin, B., Mathews-Bradshaw, B., & Siegel, S. (2010). Adolescent and young adult oncology training for health professionals: A position statement. *Journal of Clinical Oncology, 28*, 4858–4861. doi:10.1200/JCO.2010.30.5508

Keegan, T.H.M., Tao, L., DeRouen, M.C., Wu, X.-C., Prasad, P., Lynch, C.F., ... AYA HOPE Study Collaborative Group. (2014). Medical care in adolescents and young adult cancer survivors: What are the biggest access-related barriers? *Journal of Cancer Survivorship, 8*, 282–292. doi:10.1007/s11764-013-0332-4

McInally, W. (2013). Lost in transition: Child to adult cancer services for young people. *British Journal of Nursing, 22*, 1314–1318. doi:10.12968/bjon.2013.22.22.1314

Moy, B., Polite, B.N., Halpern, M.T., Stranne, S.K., Winer, E.P., Wollins, D.S., & Newman, L.A. (2011). American Society of Clinical Oncology policy statement: Opportunities in the Patient Protection and Affordable Care Act to reduce cancer care disparities. *Journal of Clinical Oncology, 29*, 3816–3824. doi:10.1200/JCO.2011.35.8903

Nathan, P.C., Hayes-Lattin, B., Sisler, J.J., & Hudson, M.M. (2011). Critical issues in transition and survivorship for adolescents and young adults with cancers. *Cancer, 117*, 2335–2341. doi:10.1002/cncr.26042

National Comprehensive Cancer Network. (2014). *NCCN Clinical Practice Guidelines in Oncology (NCCN Guidelines®): Adolescent and young adult (AYA) oncology* [v.2.2015]. Retrieved from http://www.nccn.org/professionals/physician_gls/pdf/aya.pdf

Olsen, P.R., & Harder, I. (2011). Caring for teenagers and young adults with cancer: A grounded theory study of network-focused nursing. *European Journal of Oncology Nursing, 15*, 152–159. doi:10.1016/j.ejon.2010.07.010

Seattle Children's Hospital. (n.d.). Cancer Care Unit. Retrieved from http://www
.seattlechildrens.org/clinics-programs/cancer/services/cancer-care-unit

Thomas, D.M., Seymour, J.F., O'Brien, T., Sawyer, S.M., & Ashley, D.M. (2006). Adolescent
and young adult cancer: A revolution in evolution? *Internal Medicine Journal, 36*, 302–307.
doi:10.1111/j.1445-5994.2006.01062.x

Thompson, K., Palmer, S., & Dyson, G. (2009). Adolescents and young adults: Issues in transition from active therapy into follow-up care. *European Journal of Oncology Nursing, 13*, 207–
212. doi:10.1016/j.ejon.2009.05.001

Zebrack, B., Kent, E.E., Keegan, T.H.M., Kato, I., Smith, A.W., & AYA HOPE Study Collaborative
Group. (2014). "Cancer sucks," and other ponderings by adolescent and young adult cancer survivors. *Journal of Psychosocial Oncology, 32*, 1–15. doi:10.1080/07347332.2013.855959

CHAPTER 4
Dating and Relationships

Introduction

Cancer in young adulthood has the potential to affect the establishment of romantic relationships, another key developmental milestone for this age group. Because its age range is so broad—15 to 39—young adulthood encompasses a range of relationship issues, from beginning to date to permanent partnerships and/or marriage, relationship dissolution, and even divorce. Those on the younger end of the spectrum will be challenged with much different issues than those who are older; however, at the root of this is the human need to love and be loved.

This chapter will discuss the unique challenges for young adults in terms of establishing and nurturing romantic relationships.

Young Adult Relationships

The earlier years of young adulthood are characterized by fluid relationships where sexual activity is the norm but commitment is less established (Manlove, Welti, Wildsmith, & Barry, 2014). This affects prevention of pregnancy and sexually transmitted infections because consistent use of contraceptive methods and communication about the need for both barrier and hormonal contraception (called the *dual method*, the most protective approach) are not always the norm. Data from the National Longitudinal Survey of Youth, a large representative study of young adults ages 18–26, showed that 75% of the more than 4,000 participants in a dating relationship had used some method of contraception at last intercourse, 26% had used a condom only (male controlled), 26% relied on a hormonal method (female controlled), and just 23% had used both (Manlove et al., 2011). As relationships increased in duration and level of intimacy, condom use decreased and reliance on hormonal methods increased.

While pregnancy prevention is important, social and relationship factors influence consistent condom use among young men. Factors contributing to inconsistent contraceptive use included low communication with partners, lack of predictability in relationships, and lack of regard for female sexual partners (Raine et al., 2010). In this study, engaging in unprotected intercourse was attributed to alcohol and drug use, not having condoms available, being "lost in the moment," and, for some, a decision to not use condoms. The young men had low levels of knowledge about hormonal contraception but subscribed to multiple myths about the danger of hormonal contraceptives for women. Those in committed relationships were more likely to rely on the young women to use this method, but the men were also mistrustful of their partners' adherence level and their desire for pregnancy.

This is the context in which young adults with cancer experience dating and relationships. Cancer, however, interrupts normal dating and the development of committed relationships, and young adults may experience challenges "catching up" with their peers after treatment. This can be especially difficult for young adults who experience recurrence of their cancer or those who are diagnosed with metastatic disease and may not experience reintegration with the peer group.

Nothing exists in the scholarly literature about young gay, lesbian, or bisexual (GLB) cancer survivors. This is not surprising given that very little exists in the literature about the experiences of adult GLB individuals with cancer. Even websites dedicated to GLB cancer survivors do not address the topic of young adults, and organizations for young adults with cancer (e.g., Stupid Cancer, Young Adult Cancer Canada) are silent about GLB survivors.

Cancer as Interruption

A diagnosis of cancer interrupts various aspects of life for young adults. For those in school, cancer treatment causes a gap in the usual socialization opportunities. While the young person's peer group is beginning to date and establish opposite- or same-sex attraction, the individual with cancer may miss most, if not all, of these opportunities. Cancer treatment takes place over months, and in some cases years, and these absences create significant gaps in both maturation and experiences. In addition, the young person may miss health and sexuality education in high school and instead have to seek this out from parents, siblings, or the Internet. The young person's parents may interfere; they may be overprotective and see their son or daughter as vulnerable, both physically and emotionally, and discourage their child from dating or spending time with peers. This, in turn, will prevent the young person from distancing from the parents, another developmental milestone, and establishing a sexual identity (Evan, Kaufman, Cook, & Zeltzer, 2006). The role of parents will be discussed in greater detail in Chapter 8.

Another task of this developmental stage is *identity formation*, in which individuals try to find out who they are in relation to others. They also need to get to know themselves and find value in who they are; this is termed *self-worth* or *self-esteem*. Identity and self-worth are essential components of independence and differentiation from parents. Cancer may cause obstacles to this process. For example, cancer affecting the central nervous system may affect cognition and insight, and the young person may be unable to form a unique identity because of cognitive changes. Alterations in appearance may influence how people value and judge themselves; low self-esteem may result because they do not like how they look and feel unattractive to others.

Romantic and sexual relationships are, in part, based on successful achievement of cultural and social norms of flirting and asking someone out on a date. Gaps in socialization due to illness can prevent a young person from learning the rules about these activities and limit opportunities to practice them. When treatment is over, young cancer survivors may lag behind their peers who have progressed without them. The physical effects of treatment—scars, weight loss or gain, stretch marks, amputation, hair loss—not only affect body image but also make survivors look different than their peers. This may further isolate young cancer survivors. One of the sentinel experiences of these formative years is fitting in with peers, and those who do not can be teased or ostracized. In the 21st-century world of the Internet, cyberbullying is a reality and can be devastating to anyone who is the recipient of hurtful and cruel communication on various forms of social media.

Relationship Stressors

Very little research exists on relationship issues for young adults with cancer. In a review on the topic in relation to testicular cancer survivors, Carpentier and Fortenberry (2010) noted that partner status appeared to be important for the survivors as they adapt to their experience and altered body. Specifically, the review found that men who were in a committed relationship at the time of diagnosis (and these were mostly older rather than younger adults, so extrapolation to a younger demographic may not be valid) were more successful in adapting to the physical and emotional consequences of the cancer experience. Men who were in a relationship during treatment were found to experience greater support and self-esteem and better mental health than unpartnered men. Some men reported that their relationship grew closer as a result of the cancer. However, for men in conflicted relationships, the diagnosis exacerbated problems or created new problems, and the relationship ended. For some men, the diagnosis caused a reevaluation of priorities; they were not willing to remain in a poor relationship and ended it. For those who were not partnered at the time of diagnosis, having cancer raised fears about being able to start a relationship in the future and left them with a sense of vulnerability that persisted even when a new relationship was formed.

Young adult cancer survivors may remain in relationships longer but experience greater distress when the relationship ends. This may highlight their belief that they have fewer options for starting a new relationship, so they may remain in the relationship even when it is not satisfactory. In addition, those who have undergone more intensive treatment are at greater risk for relationship difficulties and lower relationship satisfaction (Thompson, Marsland, Marshal, & Tersak, 2009).

Some literature has been published about breast cancer survivors and their relationships. Much of this literature focused on abandonment of the woman by her male partner. In an older article (Taylor-Brown, Kilpatrick, Maunsell, & Dorval, 2000), the authors found no evidence supporting the contention that the male partners of women with breast cancer leave the relationship. The evidence they found was that relationships in fact grew closer and that marital breakdown was more likely in previously conflicted relationships. Another older study (Gluhoski, Siegel, & Gorey, 1998) found mostly negative experiences among single women with breast cancer. The women in this study were pessimistic about future relationships, felt isolated with inadequate support, and were fearful of disclosing their illness to partners. Some of the women reported being rejected by their partners soon after diagnosis or living in anticipation of rejection.

The findings of a qualitative study of 15 young breast cancer survivors provided a detailed description of dating and new relationships (Kurowecki & Fergus, 2014). This study described a key challenge of life after breast cancer—"wearing my heart on my chest"—in which women experienced great emotional vulnerability about revealing their cancer history and altered body to a new sexual partner. The establishment of a new relationship was described as unfolding in a stage-like process. This involved first reclaiming the self and physical self-esteem, then starting to date and testing potential partners in their acceptance of the breast cancer, and finally experiencing self-acceptance emerging from the establishment of the new relationship.

Women described the breast cancer experience as one where trust in the body was lost and new insecurities, and worsening of old ones, changed how they saw themselves (Kurowecki & Fergus, 2014). Women recognized that they needed to find ways to cope with these physical changes and find self-acceptance and that this needed to happen before they could begin dating again. Some women who had been in a relationship at the time of diagnosis reported dissolution of that relationship, which led to feelings of abandonment. For some, the cancer created a distance between the couple and led to the breakup. Women were acutely aware of feeling "damaged" and that it might be difficult to find a new partner, and this made them feel insecure and at the same time resigned to being single for the rest of their lives. The physical changes from treatment resulted in women feeling deformed and led to comparisons with nonaffected women. This left survivors feeling that they could not measure up to "healthy" women. They also recognized that their potential infertility could affect their desirability to men who would rather be with a woman who could provide them with a family (Kurowecki & Fergus, 2014).

Acceptance of their cancer experience, altered body, and sense of self was a gradual process for the women in this study. Some of the women not only regained their sense of who they were but also felt stronger, more empowered, and more independent as a result of the cancer. Dating after cancer was, in part, dependent on this self-acceptance, and as they became more accepting, they were able to weigh the pros and cons of dating and the risks of opening themselves up to a new relationship. Dating was a process of aligning their requirements for a new partner with the reality of what potential partners existed. The women wanted someone who they thought would be able to cope with a woman affected by cancer. Men were expected to be older, with some experience of cancer, and to have their priorities established. Women were not prepared to settle for someone who would not treat them well and who would not be ready for commitment. However, they also recognized that they might only find someone who also had health issues or perhaps who was not that attractive. Online dating was a frequently used strategy to meet men because this provided the women with some control and a feeling of safety. Women were also willing to be introduced to men by friends or acquaintances (Kurowecki & Fergus, 2014).

The disclosure of the cancer (see next section) was somewhat of a test of the men's ability to accept their cancer history. The immediate response, verbally and with body language, was a test of character, and the men then needed to demonstrate genuine interest about the woman as a person. The women took time to educate potential partners about the treatments they had and prepared the men for the unveiling of the altered body by describing their scars, showing them the breast prosthesis, and slowly revealing their bodies. This was uniformly anxiety provoking and usually done with low light in the room and with the affected area covered. Men who were accepting were rewarded with greater closeness and willingness to share verbally what the woman had gone through. Women felt lucky if they found someone who was accepting, and they described these men as being special. The men who were interested in an ongoing relationship were seen to be warm, solid, unwavering, strong, and not likely to abandon them. These qualities, together with the changed values and priorities of the women, led to stronger and deeper relationships for the most part. Men who appeared disinterested in the survivor's experience of breast cancer were seen as lacking, but some women did not want to raise this as an issue that needed to be dealt with for fear of losing him and having to start dating again (Kurowecki & Fergus, 2014).

In a qualitative study of 10 women (both partnered and single) with breast cancer and 5 male partners (Holmberg, Scott, Alexy, & Fife, 2001), single women reported more anger and sadness than their partnered counterparts. These women reported little support from ex-partners, and some women stated that their ex-partners were intentionally cruel and made hurtful comments about their appearance and sexual desirability. This made some women fearful that future partners may react in the same way. Another concern of single women was how and when and how much to disclose about their cancer to new partners. This is a constant theme in the few studies of single individuals with cancer and will be discussed separately in the following pages. The partnered women noted problems with communication with their partners and changes in how they resolved conflicts following diagnosis and treatment (Holmberg et al., 2001). Participants reported protecting each other by not discussing fears about death. Male partners reported great anxiety about their wives dying and leaving them alone. Their response was to do more for their wives by helping with household chores as a way of trying to influence the outcome of the disease process. They also worried a lot and were very concerned about their wives' recovery.

In comparison, in a study of newly diagnosed partnered women with breast cancer, 42% of the couples surveyed said that the cancer had made them closer and was a growth experience. Just 6% of the couples in the study reported one of the couple feeling distanced, and only 1% reported that both members experienced distancing (Dorval et al., 2005).

Women with breast or brain cancer are less likely to be married than healthy women; however, women with other kinds of cancer are no less likely to be married. Men with cancer are more likely to be married than their healthy counterparts, but this likelihood is small (5%) (Syse, 2008). Young adults have been found to be less likely to be married than healthy people of similar age (58% vs. 64%, relative risk = 0.92, 95% confidence interval [0.85, 0.99]) (Kirchhoff, Yi, Wright, Warner, & Smith, 2012). Divorce was more likely for young adult cancer survivors, and women were more likely than men to be divorced (Kirchhoff et al., 2012). The authors of this study suggested that the stress of cancer may strain relatively new marriages that cannot overcome the physical, emotional, and financial challenges and the resultant uncertainty of living with cancer. While marriage may bring more support to young adults with cancer, newer relationships may not be resilient enough, and the additional stress of possibly raising young children and of job insecurity may prove too much for the relationship.

The risk of relationship dissolution appears to be greater if the person who is ill is a woman. Glantz et al. (2009) found a sixfold increase in relationship breakdown when the affected partner was female. They concluded that the incentive to remain in a relationship with a sick partner reflects a commitment, and women are more likely to commit to a sick male partner than vice versa.

Disclosure

Telling someone about a current or past diagnosis of cancer is regarded by almost all single cancer survivors as a sentinel and challenging task in establishing a new relationship. In a study of breast cancer survivors, 68% were afraid to disclose their cancer status to a new partner two years after completion of treatment. This dropped to 22% a year later, suggesting that perhaps it gets easier either with time or with greater distance from treatment (Ganz et al., 1996).

In Kurowecki and Fergus's (2014) study of breast cancer survivors, when and how to disclose were foremost concerns for these women. The women in this study stated that disclosure was essential before any physical contact took place, and this was viewed as a way of warning potential partners. Full disclosure was seen as a way of preventing heartbreak later on, so it had to be done early in the relationship, and the disclosure needed to be full and detailed with nothing left unsaid or hidden. The man's response to the disclosure was a test, and the women in this study were hypervigilant to not only the man's verbal response but also his facial expressions and body language.

In another study of breast cancer survivors (Gluhoski et al., 1998), the women interviewed struggled with when and how to disclose, and some were so uncomfortable doing this that they avoided new relationships. Most of this fear was based on the fear of rejection, and for some, this was based on a past experience where disclosure had resulted in a rapid end to an existing relationship. Part of the disclosure also involved informing a potential partner about the survivor's changed body and not just about the cancer. For some women, this was so scary that they would rather remain single or stay in an unsatisfactory relationship to avoid the need to disclose in the future (Holmberg et al., 2001). Carpentier, Fortenberry, Ott, Brames, and Einhorn (2011) reported similar fears among unpartnered men with testicular cancer.

How to Help the Young Adult With Cancer

How can oncology care providers guide single cancer survivors who seek assistance with fears about dating and relationships? The professional literature lacks information for the most part. Evan et al. (2006) acknowledged this silence and made suggestions based on their clinical experience. They recognized that oncology care providers need to know the context of the survivors' lives and must be aware of the developmental stages, milestones, and tasks of emerging and young adulthood and must offer treatment with this in mind. This also means recognizing when parents should not be present for sensitive discussions, such as those about sexual health, contraception, and establishment of new relationships. Parents may be overprotective of their young adult children and may consciously or unconsciously maintain dependence that ultimately prevents individuals from accomplishing the tasks of this developmental stage.

Evan et al. (2006) suggested that attaining personal control can be constructive, as this can help build self-esteem and sexual health in young adults. Many young adults have control taken away by the cancer and treatments that feel imposed, even when critically necessary. Offering choices to the young adult wherever possible may help foster confidence in decision making and give back some ownership and choice when most of it has been taken away. This may transfer into self-confidence in relationship issues and choices about whom to be sexual with or not. However, this must be associated with age-appropriate sexual health education for those who may have missed this education in high school or college.

It is important to ask, respectfully and gently, about the relationship status of young adult patients and survivors for whom we care. Neutral language, such as "partner" instead of "girlfriend" or "boyfriend" or saying "girlfriend *or* boyfriend," will help to avoid making GLB individuals feel excluded. Healthcare providers should tell patients why they are asking about their relationship status (because the care team needs to know who is there to support the patient) and show genuine interest in their response. Healthcare providers also should ask about any changes in the relationship that have occurred because of the cancer and treatment regimen and offer support and referrals where appropriate if the young adult discloses relationship stress.

If patients are not in a relationship, asking about their relationship status will offer opportunities to talk about why not, and this may open the door to talking about how they feel about themselves and their hopes and dreams for the future. It may also open the conversation to important topics such as sexuality and body image and may allow for dispelling of myths and misinformation about a variety of topics. Because many young adults are treated in the pediatric setting (see Chapter 3), relationship status may not be a part of the routine assessment. It may also be standard protocol to have one or both parents with the patient in these settings, and the medical and nursing staff may not ask questions about this to protect the privacy of the patient—and to reduce embarrassment for the parents, the patient, and themselves.

Many young adults struggle with when and how much to disclose to actual or potential romantic partners. Providing an answer to this question is challenging, but each time healthcare providers ask young adult survivors when they think is the right time, they will provide examples and anecdotal evidence that can benefit other patients.

Some young adult survivors choose to disclose up front, such as on the first date or even before the date happens. They watch for body language and facial expression in response to the disclosure and then decide if they want to see that person again. The rationale for this is that full and unconditional acceptance is the only thing they will accept, and any hesitation or suggestion of shock is an automatic rejection of the other person. The risk of this approach is that it does not allow for second thought on the part of the potential date. Most young people have never met anyone with cancer and may not even be aware that young people can have cancer. Rejecting them on the basis of an unconscious facial expression in reaction to a disclosure that is shocking is likely not fair and may mean that people who could be accepting and supportive once they have had time to get used to the idea are rejected out of hand.

Others choose to wait until the second or third date to disclose. The advantage of this approach is that there is time to see if the relationship has the potential to progress. It may also be protective for young adult survivors to disclose only when they are sure that there is potential in the relationship but before they are emotionally involved. For many survivors, disclosure is something that makes them vulnerable and requires emotional energy each and every time they say the words "I have [or had] cancer." As described earlier in this chapter, disclosure is fraught with fear for many survivors, and the fear of the response to the disclosure may prevent some young, single survivors from even contemplating dating.

People sometimes use a host of platitudes to encourage single people to date and seek out potential partners: if you don't try you won't ever know; there's somebody out there for everyone; if someone doesn't accept who you are then he or she isn't right for you anyway; there are plenty of fish in the sea. These are not helpful, particularly coming from a healthcare provider. The following questions may elicit responses that care providers can build on that are more constructive for young adults in building confidence and may even help them to "take the plunge."

- What would need to happen for you to think about going on a date?
- What scares you most about telling someone you have cancer?
- What has been your past experience with disclosing your cancer history?
- What would be the worst response to disclosing your cancer history?
- What would be the best response to disclosing your cancer history?

It may help to practice the disclosure conversation with the young adult survivor. Some people are so scared about this that they have not formulated a plan for how they would start the conversation about their cancer history. Providing them with an opportunity to practice saying the words in a safe and nonthreatening environment with someone to support and guide them may be very helpful.

In answer to the question "How much do you tell?" the following tips may be useful for young adults.

- It all depends on what you are comfortable disclosing.
- A good place to start is to state simply "I had cancer ___ months (or years) ago."
- Wait for a response. If they don't say anything immediately, don't try to fill the silence. (This is big stuff, and they may need to collect their thoughts for a few moments.)
- If they change the subject, it may mean that they aren't able to process this and you need to ask them at another time what they think or feel about your disclosure.
- If they ask you to tell them more about what happened, you can start simply and allow their questions to guide how much detail to give. (Katz, 2014, pp. 94–95)

Romantic Partners of Young Adults With Cancer

Support and love from a partner has both tangible and intangible benefits for young adults with cancer. As with cancer survivors of all ages, partner support is essential for both instrumental day-to-day living and, perhaps even more importantly, for emotional support and encouragement. Like many other issues for young adults, literature specific to this age group is lacking. Emerging adults are unlikely to have partners involved in their care, and because the vast majority of cancer survivors are older than 60 years of age, attention has been focused on that population. The studies cited in this chapter all had younger participants; however, it is difficult to identify specifics about those on the younger end of the spectrum, and caution should be used when interpreting the findings and conclusions unless they specifically mention age as a variable.

Outside of the context of cancer, the kind of support provided by a partner has a significant impact on life in general. A partner who is nurturing and provides emotional as well as tangible support is beneficial. A partner who is negative and critical or controlling does not enhance life satisfaction for the other. When partners help each other, the relationship improves and self-improvement is more likely to occur (Overall, Fletcher, & Simpson, 2010).

Impact of Cancer on the Caregiving Partner or Spouse

Cancer causes a major disruption to all facets of life. Young adults with cancer often have to take a break from work or school to undergo treatment, and side effects of treatment may necessitate taking a break from the usual roles that the person with cancer plays at home. Child care, household tasks, shopping, and general caregiving of the family that is often performed by one individual, frequently a woman, may now fall to the partner or spouse. When the person with cancer is the major earner in the family, household income may fall, especially if the person does not have paid sick time from work. This can cause great upheaval and anxiety.

In a review of spousal caregiving (Li & Loke, 2013), female partners had higher levels of negative experiences than male partners when taking care of their spouse or partner with cancer. Women reported poorer mental and physical health, as well as lower health-related quality of life. Women were also more likely to experience less satisfaction with life in general and decreased marital satisfaction than men. Partners, like survivors, often have unmet needs along the cancer trajectory. It is known that partners may experience levels of distress that are higher than those of cancer survivors (Bowman, Rose, & Deimling, 2006) and may ignore their own needs in favor of supporting and caring for their partner. Turner et al. (2013) studied the health and well-being in partners or close family members of long-term (more than five years) cancer survivors. Most of the respondents indicated that they had moved on from the experience with an average of only 2.7 unmet needs out of a possible 34. They wanted information about familial cancer risk and help managing their own fear of cancer recurring in their partner or spouse. Their levels of anxiety and depression were the same as population norms, except for a small proportion (10%) who were highly anxious with many unmet needs. Respondents reported positive gains, with two-thirds stating that they had a greater appreciation of life after their partner's cancer experience, and 40% felt that they had become stronger people as a result. This personal growth has also been described by other researchers and will be described in greater detail in Chapter 10.

The changes caused by cancer for couples have also been studied. In one study (Drabe, Wittmann, Zwahlen, Büchi, & Jenewein, 2013), 57.9% of survivors and 55.5% of their partners reported positive changes only. Negative changes only were reported by a minority of those studies (3.8% of survivors and 8.6% of their partners). Approximately 10% of survivors and partners reported a mix of positive and negative changes. Both male and female partners who experienced negative changes in their relationship also reported lower quality of life and higher levels of anxiety and depression. Change in the dyadic relationship was noted by the majority of respondents in this study (71.3% of survivors and 74.6% of their partners); however, female partners experienced negative changes more frequently than male partners (Drabe et al., 2013).

Male partners or spouses may be considered in a unique position given the Western norms of women providing most of the supportive care in relationships, although this may be different among young adults who have been raised in dual-income families and more egalitarian households. Once again, little research has been done on young male partners of women with cancer, but some studies have addressed the specific experiences of male partners of younger women with breast cancer.

In a study of older male partners of women with breast cancer, stereotypical male responses included protecting and caring for the women and trying to enhance their coping by being positive (Lopez, Copp, & Molassiotis, 2012). The men in this study changed their lifestyle to support their wives or partners and admitted to needing support themselves but finding it difficult to ask for help, especially from other men. The men were the ones to tell family and friends about their partner's cancer diagnosis and were also involved in finding information about the disease and suggesting alternative treatments, particularly complementary and alternative treatments. They were unprepared to take on the household tasks that their partners used to do but eventually got used to it, often between six and nine months after their partner's diagnosis. Some men took off time from work while their partner underwent treatment, which then caused worry about financial matters. Emotional side effects included fear about losing their spouse or partner and fear of the unknown. This occurred in the context of lack of social support and limited social contacts making them vulnerable to emotional distress with little ability to ask for help.

In a study of male spouses of breast cancer survivors (Duggleby, Doell, Cooper, Thomas, & Ghosh, 2014), predictors of their quality of life were age (older men had better quality of life than younger men), hope, self-efficacy, feelings of guilt, and the quality of life of the women with breast cancer. The authors of this study suggested that interventions targeting hope and self-efficacy and addressing feelings of guilt in men may improve the quality of life in the husbands of women with breast cancer.

In a study of partners of long-term survivors of gynecologic cancer (Stafford & Judd, 2010), 48.5% had at least one unmet need. However, the respondents had generally low levels of depression (8.8%) and anxiety (10.3%). If the partner perceived the relationship with the cancer survivor as being poor, he experienced greater anxiety. Somewhat surprisingly, the men in this study did not experience altered sexual satisfaction even though their partners reported vaginal changes.

How to Help the Partner or Spouse of the Young Adult With Cancer

It is important to pay attention to the supportive care needs of the patient and the partner or spouse as individuals and also the couple as a dyad. Given that young adult patients may have young children of their own, the resulting responsibilities and stress on the partner or spouse may be significant. It is not routine practice to assess the health and coping of partners or spouses, but if they are present for appointments, asking them how they are coping may identify those who are struggling or feeling overwhelmed. In their review of hidden morbidities among spousal caregivers, Li and Loke (2013) noted that the evidence suggests interventions for young adult partners or spouses should focus on improving empathetic listening and communication, improving the ability of the couple and the spouse or partner to cope with what is happening, and helping the couple to understand each other's needs.

Referral of spouses or partners to psychosocial clinicians is an obvious suggestion, but one that might be met with refusal by already overextended partners or spouses who are trying to find the time for the basic activities of daily life as well as supporting their partner with cancer instrumentally and emotionally. However, receiving supportive care and encouragement can be of benefit to struggling partners or spouses. This might be particularly important for men, who tend to avoid asking for help. Duggleby et al. (2014) suggested that supportive care for partners or spouses, including interventions to foster hope, increase self-efficacy, and decrease guilt, may be of particular benefit.

Couples often have difficulty talking about sensitive topics (such as sex) with each other. Young couples with a short relationship history may have a particularly difficult time when faced with the stresses inherent in the cancer experience. The following are some suggestions to give to patients and partners for having a difficult conversation.

- Don't make assumptions about what your partner is thinking or feeling.
- Talk in "I" statements and allow your partner to talk for and about himself or herself.
- Don't talk about sexual problems in bed or while naked.
- Listen (*really listen*) to what your partner has to say.
- Validate (I hear what you're saying) instead of fighting (no, I don't!).
- Think about writing down what you want to say in a letter.
- Schedule time to talk about what you've written.
- Some couples need help talking about sensitive topics. Consider seeing a therapist or counselor. (Katz, 2014, pp. 117–118)

In a study of couples of all ages evaluating a couple-based intervention where one of the couple was newly diagnosed with cancer (McMahon, Gremore, Cella, & Sher, 2014), participants reported that the intervention provided a safe place for them to talk about sensitive topics that they might have avoided, as well as validated their feelings. The six sessions covered topics such as working as a team and communicating with healthcare providers, reallocating household tasks, improving couple communication, encouraging supportive behaviors, adopting effective coping strategies, and discussing sexuality. While formal programs covering these topics may not be possible for all healthcare settings, these issues may form the basis of a formal assessment of couple coping that could be performed at specific times during the cancer journey. Examples of questions that can be asked are

- How are you coping as a couple with one of you having cancer?
- What are the differences in your coping styles, and how has this affected your relationship?
- What do you do when you encounter feelings that you have never felt before?
- Who is supporting you as the partner/spouse?
- What is your greatest worry at the moment?
- Is there anything you want your partner or spouse to know that you have not been able to tell him or her?

Caregivers also can complete the National Comprehensive Cancer Network® Distress Thermometer (see Chapter 10) to formally identify areas of concern.

Support groups for partners of young adults with cancer may exist in larger communities, and events such as Stupid Cancer's CancerCon and the Young Adult Cancer Canada annual conference encourage participation by partners and spouses and also have sessions specifically for them. See http://cancercon.org and www.youngadultcancer.ca/our-programs for information about these two programs.

Conclusion

Establishing romantic relationships is an important task of young adulthood and one that can be interrupted or postponed by cancer. After cancer, young adults often are changed individuals and sometimes are out of sync with their peer group, resulting in multiple challenges in this important aspect of life. Oncology care providers are often older than their young adult patients and can find it awkward to talk about dating and relationships when their own experience of this is in the distant past. However, healthcare providers have a responsibility to support young adult survivors in recovering both physically and emotionally from the side effects of treatment. Offering guidance in this realm of their lives after cancer is an essential part of providing holistic care.

The paucity of evidence on the issues affecting the partners and spouses of young adults with cancer limits care providers' knowledge of how these young men and women are affected when their partner is diagnosed with cancer. How same-sex partners are affected is not articulated at all in the literature, and assumptions cannot be made based on the limited evidence for older, heterosexual individuals. This area is ripe for research and discovery.

References

Bowman, K.F., Rose, J.H., & Deimling, G.T. (2006). Appraisal of the cancer experience by family members and survivors in long-term survivorship. *Psycho-Oncology, 15,* 834–845. doi:10.1002/pon.1039

Carpentier, M.Y., & Fortenberry, J.D. (2010). Romantic and sexual relationships, body image, and fertility in adolescent and young adult testicular cancer survivors: A review of the literature. *Journal of Adolescent Health, 47,* 115–125. doi:10.1016/j.jadohealth.2010.04.005

Carpentier, M.Y., Fortenberry, J.D., Ott, M.A., Brames, M.J., & Einhorn, L.H. (2011). Perceptions of masculinity and self-image in adolescent and young adult testicular cancer survivors: Implications for romantic and sexual relationships. *Psycho-Oncology, 20,* 738–745. doi:10.1002/pon.1772

Dorval, M., Guay, S., Mondor, M., Mâsse, B., Falardeau, M., Robidoux, A., … Maunsell, E. (2005). Couples who get closer after breast cancer: Frequency and predictors in a prospective investigation. *Journal of Clinical Oncology, 23,* 3588–3596. doi:10.1200/JCO.2005.01.628

Drabe, N., Wittmann, L., Zwahlen, D., Büchi, S., & Jenewein, J. (2013). Changes in close relationships between cancer patients and their partners. *Psycho-Oncology, 22,* 1344–1352. doi:10.1002/pon.3144

Duggleby, W., Doell, H., Cooper, D., Thomas, R., & Ghosh, S. (2014). The quality of life of male spouses of women with breast cancer: Hope, self-efficacy, and perceptions of guilt. *Cancer Nursing, 37,* E28–E35. doi:10.1097/NCC.0b013e31827ca807

Evan, E.E., Kaufman, M., Cook, A.B., & Zeltzer, L.K. (2006). Sexual health and self-esteem in adolescents and young adults with cancer. *Cancer, 107,* 1672–1679. doi:10.1002/cncr.22101

Ganz, P.A., Coscarelli, A., Fred, C., Kahn, B., Polinsky, M.L., & Petersen, L. (1996). Breast cancer survivors: Psychosocial concerns and quality of life. *Breast Cancer Research and Treatment, 38,* 183–199. doi:10.1007/BF01806673

Glantz, M.J., Chamberlain, M.C., Liu, Q., Hsieh, C-C., Edwards, K.R., Van Horn, A., & Recht, L. (2009). Gender disparity in the rate of partner abandonment in patients with serious medical illness. *Cancer, 115,* 5237–5242. doi:10.1002/cncr.24577

Gluhoski, V.L., Siegel, K., & Gorey, E. (1998). Unique stressors experienced by unmarried women with breast cancer. *Journal of Psychosocial Oncology, 15*(3–4), 173–183. doi:10.1300/J077v15n03_08

Holmberg, S.K., Scott, L.L., Alexy, W., & Fife, B.L. (2001). Relationship issues of women with breast cancer. *Cancer Nursing, 24,* 53–60. doi:10.1097/00002820-200102000-00009

Katz, A. (2014). *This should not be happening: Young adults with cancer.* Pittsburgh, PA: Hygeia Media.

Kirchhoff, A.C., Yi, J., Wright, J., Warner, E.L., & Smith, K.R. (2012). Marriage and divorce among young adult cancer survivors. *Journal of Cancer Survivorship, 6,* 441–450. doi:10.1007/s11764-012-0238-6

Kurowecki, D., & Fergus, K.D. (2014). Wearing my heart on my chest: Dating, new relationships, and the reconfiguration of self-esteem after breast cancer. *Psycho-Oncology, 23,* 52–64. doi:10.1002/pon.3370

Li, W., & Loke, A.Y. (2013). A spectrum of hidden morbidities among spousal caregivers for patients with cancer, and differences between the genders: A review of the literature. *European Journal of Oncology Nursing, 17,* 578–587. doi:10.1016/j.ejon.2013.01.007

Lopez, V., Copp, G., & Molassiotis, A. (2012). Male caregivers of patients with breast and gynecologic cancer: Experiences from caring for their spouses and partners. *Cancer Nursing, 35,* 402–410. doi:10.1097/NCC.0b013e318231daf0

Manlove, J., Welti, K., Barry, M., Peterson, K., Schelar, E., & Wildsmith, E. (2011). Relationship characteristics and contraceptive use among young adults. *Perspectives on Sexual and Reproductive Health, 43,* 119–128. doi:10.1363/4311911

Manlove, J., Welti, K., Wildsmith, E., & Barry, M. (2014). Relationship types and contraceptive use within young adult dating relationships. *Perspectives on Sexual and Reproductive Health, 46,* 41–50. doi:10.1363/46e0514

McMahon, M.E., Gremore, T.M., Cella, D., & Sher, T.G. (2014). Partners empowered: A couple-based intervention for newly diagnosed cancer. *Psycho-Oncology, 23,* 832–834. doi:10.1002/pon.3490

Overall, N.C., Fletcher, G.J.O., & Simpson, J.A. (2010). Helping each other grow: Romantic partner support, self-improvement, and relationship quality. *Personality and Social Psychology Bulletin, 36,* 1496–1513. doi:10.1177/0146167210383045

Raine, T.R., Gard, J.C., Boyer, C.B., Haider, S., Brown, B.A., Hernandez, F.A.R., & Harper, C.C. (2010). Contraceptive decision-making in sexual relationships: Young men's experiences, attitudes and values. *Culture, Health and Sexuality, 12,* 373–386. doi:10.1080/13691050903524769

Stafford, L., & Judd, F. (2010). Partners of long-term gynaecologic cancer survivors: Psychiatric morbidity, psychosexual outcomes and supportive care needs. *Gynecologic Oncology, 118,* 268–273. doi:10.1016/j.ygyno.2010.05.019

Syse, A. (2008). Does cancer affect marriage rates? *Journal of Cancer Survivorship, 2,* 205–214. doi:10.1007/s11764-008-0062-1

Taylor-Brown, J., Kilpatrick, M., Maunsell, E., & Dorval, M. (2000). Partner abandonment of women with breast cancer: Myth or reality? *Cancer Practice, 8,* 160–164. doi:10.1046/j.1523-5394.2000.84004.x

Thompson, A.L., Marsland, A.L., Marshal, M.P., & Tersak, J.M. (2009). Romantic relationships of emerging adult survivors of childhood cancers. *Psycho-Oncology, 18,* 767–774. doi:10.1002/pon.1471

Turner, D., Adams, E., Boulton, M., Harrison, S., Khan, N., Rose, P., … Watson, E.K. (2013). Partners and close family members of long-term cancer survivors: Health status, psychosocial well-being and unmet supportive care needs. *Psycho-Oncology, 22,* 12–19. doi:10.1002/pon.2050

CHAPTER 5
Sexuality and Contraception

Introduction

Despite the role that sexuality plays in the lives of young adults, an insufficient amount of literature exists on the topic in this population. Some attention has been paid to this for childhood cancer survivors, particularly in the area of sexual development in the aftermath of treatment; however, the issues for young adult survivors are different. Young adulthood, the years between ages 15 and 39, is a time of sexual exploration and experimentation. It is also a time when romantic relationships are formed and cemented, as described in Chapter 4.

Cancer and its treatments profoundly affect sexuality and sexual functioning. It is important to differentiate between sexuality and sexual functioning or activity. In short, *sexuality* is a broad concept encompassing sexual self-identity as men or women, sexual orientation, gender roles, sexual thoughts and fantasies, and erotic triggers. Sexual activity or functioning, alone or with a partner, is the enactment of some or all aspects of one's sexuality. It is also important to note that fertility and sexuality are not the same and should not be conceptualized as similar. They should be discussed in an age-appropriate manner as separate and distinct areas of impact of cancer treatment.

This chapter will describe the little evidence that exists about sexuality in the young adult population, including information about the limited interventions for sexual problems after cancer. The final section will address the need for contraception for young men and women in this age group. This chapter aims to provide readers with the tools to understand the unique needs of young adults with cancer as they relate to sexuality in a broad context; these needs are often unmet and are the source of distress for those affected.

Healthy Sexual Functioning

Sexual functioning is dependent, in part, on intact vascular and neurologic structures. It also relies on healthy endocrine function for the production of sex hormones that initiate the maturation of the sex organs (breasts, vulva and vagina, uterus, and ovaries in women; testicles and penis in men), as well as other physical signs of sexual maturity such as body hair and the typical male or female body shape. The brain is involved as well; important aspects of sexual functioning such as sexual desire and the subjective experience of arousal and orgasm are directly related to interpretation in the brain.

The understanding of the human sexual response cycle is largely based on the pioneering work of Masters and Johnson and others such as Helen Singer Kaplan, who was a student of theirs. Masters and Johnson (1966) described the human sexual response cycle as being a linear, four-stage process. These four stages—excitement, plateau, orgasm, and resolution—are reflective of physical processes in which blood flows into and out of the sexual organs under the influence of nerve impulses. Excitement and plateau are essentially stages of vasocongestion. Orgasm comprises contractions of the pelvic floor muscles in both men and women, the uterus in women, and the prostate in men. The resolution phase is a result of the return of blood from the sexual organs into the general circulation.

Kaplan (1979) introduced the idea of a cognitive component in her three-stage model. The stages she described were desire, excitement, and orgasm. Desire is an important cognitive and emotional event that is interpreted by many as the first stage of her model. However, Kaplan never intended her model to be linear; she saw it as a circular model with three distinct and independent phases. In her view, excitement can be experienced as a purely physical sensation of arousal without first experiencing desire.

A more recent model conceptualized by Basson (2005) described a unique perspective of the female sexual response cycle. In this circular model, desire is depicted as being reactive to physical and mental stimuli rather than spontaneous in onset. The model also includes social and emotional factors such as the nature of the relationship, as well as contextual and motivating factors that may not be sexual at all but rather situated in purely practical considerations of safety and shelter. This model is meaningful for women in relationships who experience lack of sexual interest (libido), as it removes the expectation that they need to feel desire in order to be sexual and allows them to consider the many reasons why women are sexual outside of their own desire or lack thereof.

Developmental Aspects

Developmental tasks for young adults include creating a sexual identity, establishing romantic and sexual relationships, and exploring sexual preferences and practices (Morgan, Davies, Palmer, & Plaster, 2010). Cancer alters this, but it does not remove these important tasks forever; young adults with cancer must still negotiate these tasks while at the same time dealing with the aftermath of treatment that may profoundly affect critical aspects of their sexuality. Cancer at this stage of life is completely unexpected, and young adults have little life experience to draw on to cope with this (Bakewell & Volker, 2005).

For some young adults, sexual identity is not yet established, and opportunities to explore are interrupted or delayed by the cancer. They may fall out of sequence with their peers and find it difficult to rejoin their peer group in social activities or developmental milestones, such as serious romantic or sexual relationships. A fuller discussion of dating and relationships can be found in Chapter 4. Having cancer may affect independence from parents by requiring young adults to remain at home or to return home after having lived independently. This can hinder their ability to date or engage in sexual activity.

It can also be extremely difficult for younger cancer survivors to talk about sexuality with parents or healthcare providers who represent authority figures (Kelly, 2013). Sexuality can become a silent concern, and this is of particular importance if the survivor is gay, lesbian, bisexual, or transgender and not "out" to parents or healthcare providers. Assumptions of heterosexuality in any discussion or assessment of the survivor will further alienate the young person.

Sexual Side Effects of Treatment

All cancer treatments have the potential to affect sexuality because of the global nature of the phenomenon of sexuality, comprising not only physical functioning but also emotional and social issues. Cancer treatment is commonly multimodal, and survivors will bear the effects of some or all of the treatments they have had.

Surgery

Surgical removal of sexual organs such as the breasts, testes, prostate, uterus and uterine tubes, cervix, or vulva may result in significant sexual morbidity. Given the need for intact blood and nerve supply for healthy sexual functioning described previously, damage to blood and nerve supply to sexual organs may significantly alter functioning even if the organs themselves are not removed. However, surgery to any part of the body may result in sexual functioning alterations. For example, scarring can lead to body image issues so that the individual does not want to appear naked in front of a partner. Functional alterations to joints and limbs from amputation can make sexual intercourse difficult. Cognitive challenges after surgery to the brain may result in the individual experiencing difficulties meeting potential partners. Damage to the pituitary gland from surgery (or radiation) can lead to hormonal deficits that affect sexual development and functioning.

Radiation

Radiation causes damage to small blood vessels that supply tissues, including mucous membranes in the genital area and mouth. For women, this causes atrophy and pain when the genital area is touched during sexual play, and penetration may not be possible due to pain. Bleeding also may occur, which can be frightening for women who fear recurrence and may associate bleeding as a sign of the cancer's return. In extreme cases, the vagina itself may become obstructed by scar tissue or adhesions, and penetration may not be possible. This also has ramifications for well-woman care because it may not be possible for the woman to have a pelvic examination or Pap test. A dry mouth makes kissing and oral sex uncomfortable or painful for both men and women and, for some survivors or their partner, not enjoyable or even possible.

The damage from radiation to nerves and blood vessels supplying the sexual organs in both men and women may affect arousal. In men, this manifests as difficulties with achieving and maintaining erection secondary to damage to the nerves that are involved in erections. In women, it may decrease vaginal or vulvar lubrication during the arousal phase of the sexual response cycle, resulting in dryness and pain. Radiation damage is progressive, and effects may be seen long after treatment is over, thus categorizing these sexual changes as late effects of treatment (Incrocci & Jensen, 2013).

Chemotherapy

Chemotherapy has a profound effect on sexual functioning for women (Jankowska, 2013). Many chemotherapy agents result in premature aging of the ovaries, causing early menopause, or it may lead to abrupt ovarian failure. Both of these phenomena are associated with the signs and symptoms of menopause: vaginal dryness, loss of libido, and hot flashes. Chemotherapy is also associated with hair loss, including loss of eyebrows, eyelashes, and pubic hair. This may make the woman feel unattractive and is distressing for many. Vaginal and vulvar dryness secondary to ovarian failure can cause daily discomfort, as well as significant pain with sexual touch or penetration. This further exacerbates lack of interest in sex. Rosenberg et al. (2014) found that fatigue, vaginal pain, and poor body image contribute to sexual dysfunction in women who received chemotherapy and that sexual interest in particular is affected by weight gain, vaginal pain, and poor body image. Chemotherapy causes emotional issues as well. For example, the loss of fertility after chemotherapy may be associated with loss of femininity, and this may affect the woman's sexual self-esteem (Krychman & Millheiser, 2013).

Less is known about the sexual side effects of chemotherapy on men. Chemotherapy combined with surgery or radiation in the treatment of testicular cancer appears to increase the incidence of erectile, ejaculatory, and sexual desire problems (Kim et al., 2012). Because of the use of multimodality treatments, it is difficult to ascribe sexual side effects to chemotherapy alone. It is suggested that some men experience loss of libido and erectile difficulties during the period of active chemotherapy, and then some recovery occurs between cycles (Breukink & Donovan, 2013). In male survivors of lymphoma, chemotherapy is associated with an increased incidence of sexual problems (Arden-Close, Eiser, & Pacey, 2011).

Issues by Cancer Type

Breast Cancer

Sexual issues related to breast cancer are specific to the type of treatment that the woman has received. Mastectomy with or without reconstruction is known to cause body image issues of greater magnitude than breast-conserving treatment (lumpectomy plus radiation) (Rosenberg et al., 2012). This may be particularly important to younger women.

Body image is a multifaceted phenomenon that is highly subjective in how women view themselves and their place in society (Boquiren, Esplen, Wong, Toner, & Warner, 2013). It is suggested that women who internalize gender roles and beliefs report greater shame and decreased adaptation to an altered body after breast cancer. Breasts represent femininity, and the loss of one or both has great symbolic meaning to many women. Despite satisfaction with the aesthetics of reconstructive surgery, some women still have body image disturbances. This may be because despite the normal appearance, the loss of a breast represents the loss of wholeness and functionality (Fang, Shu, & Chang, 2013). During the time of diagnosis and treatment decision making, women may not consider the effects of treatment on body image and sexuality. The diagnosis poses a life-or-death crisis, and most women are consumed with thoughts of survival rather than aesthetics.

For women who choose bilateral mastectomy in an attempt to prevent contralateral breast cancer in the future or for aesthetic reasons, the loss of both breasts can have a profound impact on sexual feelings beyond body image. After reconstructive surgery, the affected breast does not look or feel like the woman's original breast. Importantly, after reconstruction, the "new" breast will not respond to sexual stimulation the way the "precancer" breast did. This is a source of distress for many women who are often not prepared for the loss of erotic potential after reconstruction. Women may choose reconstruction to try to feel normal and to appear normal to their partner and others, as well as to complete their cancer journey (Beesley, Ullmer, Holcombe, & Salmon, 2012).

Many women complain that after lumpectomy, depending on the amount of tissue removed, they have difficulty finding a comfortable and well-fitting bra or swimsuit. This is a practical issue that might not be discussed with patients, who may think that breast-conserving surgery will leave their breast the same as before. The same concerns apply after women have a mastectomy and have to wear a breast prosthesis either permanently or while waiting for delayed reconstruction. Body image also can be affected by the tattoos necessary for radiation therapy in addition to the skin changes from the radiation itself. One of the most common side effects of radiation is fatigue, and when this is coupled with child care, women often do not have time for anything, especially thinking about sex, nevermind participating.

Interpreting the results of studies on the association between body image and sexuality after breast cancer surgery is challenging. Markopoulos et al. (2009) reported that while more than 75% of women who had breast-conserving surgery were satisfied with their body image, 42% were dissatisfied with their sex life. Among those who had reconstruction after mastectomy, 81% reported satisfaction with their sex life, 75% said the surgery did not affect their sex life, and 68% reported no decrease in their "sexual willingness."

Endocrine treatment to prevent recurrence in younger women usually involves the prescription of a selective estrogen receptor modulator such as tamoxifen. This medication has side effects that may affect sexual functioning, including hot flashes that disrupt sleep, causing fatigue. Tamoxifen also is associated with loss of libido and, for some, vaginal dryness or atrophy, causing dyspareunia (Jankowska, 2013). Schover (2014) noted that tamoxifen can have a weak estrogenic effect on vaginal tissues and therefore may be beneficial when amenorrhea occurs after chemotherapy.

In a large study (N = 1,965) of women with breast cancer describing frequency of sexual activity, sexual response, and sexual satisfaction, changes were attributed to many causes, including menopausal changes such as vaginal dryness, pain, fatigue, and weight gain and other body image issues, as well as psychological distress (Ussher, Perz, & Gilbert, 2012). All these symptoms may be associated with problems, perceived or real, in the partner relationship. In a study from France (Brédart et al., 2011), lack of sexual activity or sexual dissatisfaction was associated with a feeling of emotional separation from the partner. For women who remained sexually active, lower frequency of sex, decreased sexual pleasure, or higher sexual discomfort was associated with emotional distance from the partner (Brédart et al., 2011). If recurrence of the cancer occurs, the need for physical connection within the couple remains. In one study of women with recurrence (Andersen, 2009), while frequency of sexual activity decreased because intercourse was too difficult or impossible, the frequency of kissing increased. Little research exists on sexuality and sexual functioning in women with recurrent or metastatic breast cancer.

Gynecologic Cancer

As with breast cancer, the sexual consequences after gynecologic cancer are multifaceted and dependent on treatment type. The more radical the surgery, the greater the sexual problems; the addition of adjuvant radiation and/or chemotherapy also increases sexual morbidity (Carter, Stabile, Gunn, & Sonoda, 2013). With novel surgical techniques such as laparoscopic surgery, sentinel lymph node mapping, and robotic surgery, it is theorized that sexual consequences will decrease. Removal of the ovaries in younger women forces them into a state of surgical menopause; the symptoms of this are widely recognized as being worse than natural menopause (Ratner, Foran, Schwartz, & Minkin, 2010). However, for younger women who menstruate after treatment, suggesting normal hormonal functioning, a return to healthy sexual functioning has been noted (Campos et al., 2012). A small study comparing women with cervical cancer treated with either surgery or radiation therapy found that those who had radiation experienced worse sexual functioning that extended for more than five years after treatment (Frumovitz et al., 2005). This is supported by another study suggesting that surgery with radiation resulted in lower quality of life and decreased frequency of sexual activity, but similar rates of sexual pleasure when compared to women treated with surgery and chemotherapy (Greimel, Winter, Kapp, & Haas, 2009). However, women with early-stage cervical cancer have reported sexual recovery six months after treatment and similar function as women with benign and precancerous conditions (Juraskova, Butow, Bonner, Robertson, & Sharpe, 2013).

In a systematic review of sexual concerns in gynecologic cancer survivors, Abbott-Anderson and Kwekkeboom (2012) reported physical and psychological problems. In the physical domain, changes in the vagina (shortening and narrowing coupled with tissue atrophy), resultant pain with intercourse, and decreased frequency of sexual activity were common. In the psychological realm, loss of libido, altered body image, and anxiety about sexual performance dominated. These all had an impact on the women's ability to maintain previous sexual roles, leading to emotional distancing from the partner and the partner experiencing an altered level of sexual interest as a result (Abbott-Anderson & Kwekkeboom, 2012). Male partners often feel out of control of the situation after the diagnosis of cancer. They also may feel guilty about wanting to be sexual with the woman and struggle to maintain an emotional connection with her, and relationship discord may result

(Ratner et al., 2010). On the other hand, a study of young women with ovarian cancer treated with chemotherapy found that couple functioning was stronger post-treatment (Gershenson et al., 2007).

Body image may be affected after surgery for gynecologic cancer. Abdominal hysterectomy generally leaves a scar on the abdomen, whereas radiation therapy to treat cervical cancer is internal and does not leave a visible scar. In a study of women after various treatments for this kind of cancer (Sekse, Gjengedal, & Råheim, 2013), participants described having to learn to live within an altered body. They stated that they had to work to regain confidence in their bodies and once again feel in control of their bodies. After surgery, the women in this study reported feeling empty and experiencing sexual changes. Vaginal dryness caused painful intercourse, making what was once a pleasurable activity problematic. The women reported lack of desire for sex that persisted more than five years after completion of treatment (Sekse et al., 2013).

How the woman sees herself as a sexual being, called *sexual self-schema*, may be an important factor in eventual recovery. Carpenter, Andersen, Fowler, and Maxwell (2009) found that women with a positive sexual self-schema were more resilient to the side effects of treatment for gynecologic cancer. Conversely, those with a negative view of their sexual selves were reluctant to resume sexual activity after treatment, were distressed by sexual problems, and were avoidant of sexual activity. They also experienced negative mood and views of themselves.

Testicular Cancer

Testicular cancer is the most common cancer in young men, and the centrality of the testes in both the physical and psychological development of masculine self-image cannot be ignored. Treatment for testicular cancer— surgery, radiation, and/or chemotherapy—leaves visible scars as well as a significant psychological impact. When testicular cancer occurs in young men who are developing their sexual self-identity, delays in achieving social and sexual maturation are possible. The impact on young men who are not yet in stable romantic relationships cannot be underestimated.

A qualitative study of men younger than age 34 with testicular cancer described four themes (Carpentier, Fortenberry, Ott, Brames, & Einhorn, 2011). First, embarrassment about finding a lump in the testicle led to delays in seeking medical treatment. The men reported that having cancer made them feel different from their peers. This, in turn, made them feel as though they were damaged goods. The final theme was that disclosing the diagnosis to others was difficult. The embarrassment related to seeking help resulted in denial of the presence of the symptom; some men only sought help under pressure from their partner. Encountering female healthcare providers made the embarrassment even more acute. The cancer experience profoundly affected these young men; they felt different from their healthy friends and believed that no one else could understand what they were going through or had experienced. For those who were partnered at the time of diagnosis, the cancer experience enriched their romantic relationship and made them appreciate the relationship more. However, single men were worried about how the diagnosis might affect future romantic relationships, particularly because they felt changed by the cancer and did not know how this would affect future partners. The physical side effects of treatment (e.g., hair loss, surgical scars, the physical loss of the testicle) contributed to the feeling of being damaged. The loss of the testicle in particular led to feelings of vulnerability, uncertainty about masculinity, and feeling incomplete. Vulnerability extended to fears about cancer in the other testicle. The profundity of the experience extended into recovery and survivorship, where partnered men reported hesitation about engaging in sexual activity again, and some even delayed doing so because they felt unsure about themselves. Disclosure of the cancer was difficult for many, particularly for unpartnered men who had significant concerns about the timing of disclosure to potential partners. For some, this uncertainty extended into whether they could have future relationships at all, given their history. Another aspect of disclosure for survivors is telling other men about their history of testicular cancer. Some men responded with jokes that were hurtful, even long after treatment. However, some survivors became advocates for screening and overcame their fear of disclosure (Carpentier et al., 2011).

Global sexual concerns were reported in a case-control study of young men with testicular cancer (Kim et al., 2012). Compared to age-matched controls, men with a history of testicular cancer had lower sex drive, poorer erections, and problems with ejaculation. In a review of the literature, Carpentier et al. (2011) noted that sexual problems, mainly related to erectile and ejaculatory function, were common. The testicles play an important role in masculine identity, sexual function, fertility, and romantic relationships. In addition, the presence of a romantic partner at the time of diagnosis and treatment was critical for long-term adjustment. Disclosure issues dominated for those who were not romantically involved at the time of diagnosis (Carpentier et al., 2011).

Lymphoma

Young adults may experience hematologic cancers such as Hodgkin lymphoma, non-Hodgkin lymphoma, and leukemia. The conditioning treatment prior to bone marrow or stem cell transplantation can have profound effects on sexuality. In a study of young women with Hodgkin lymphoma (Eeltink et al., 2013), 39% reported one or more sexual problems that were long lasting and from which they had not recovered. Sexual problems encompassed a broad range including lack of desire, arousal problems, lack of lubrication, decreased satisfaction, and pain. Lack of libido and problems with arousal were the top two problems identified. In another study of Hodgkin lymphoma survivors of both genders, sexual functioning was problematic at baseline and was worse for those with more advanced disease (Behringer et al., 2013). Functioning improved after treatment and eventually normalized for those with early-stage disease. For those with more advanced disease, sexual functioning improved after treatment but did not reach levels suggestive of healthy sexual functioning. Overall, 50% of study participants did not report severe sexual dysfunction. For survivors who were more than seven years out from treatment, significant sexual problems as compared to healthy controls were noted in another study (Recklitis, Varela, Ng, Mauch, & Bober, 2010). Almost 55% of the survivors reported decreased sexual activity compared to controls, and 41.5% reported decreased libido. However, survivors reported overall satisfaction with their sex lives. In a study of men with Hodgkin and non-Hodgkin lymphoma (Arden-Close et al., 2011), 20%–54% experienced sexual problems. Chemotherapy, relapse, and low testosterone were associated with sexual dysfunction. Emotional distress was linked to decreased sexual activity. In this study, younger men experienced fewer sexual problems than their older counterparts.

Colorectal Cancer

Colorectal cancer treatment generally is multimodal and differs according to the anatomic level of disease in the gastrointestinal tract. Colon cancer will have different sexual effects compared to anal or rectal cancer. Sexual side effects of surgery directly relate to the amount of nerve damage that occurs during the surgical procedure; nerve preservation is possible for some cancers but is largely dependent on the skill of the surgeon. The lower the location of the cancer in the colon, the greater the risk of sexual dysfunction after surgery (Donovan, Thompson, & Hoffe, 2010). The need for an ostomy, either temporary or permanent, has a significant impact on body image. Fears related to the integrity of the ostomy bag during sexual activity also may have a negative impact.

In a review of the physical and psychological effects of treatment for colorectal cancer on sexual functioning, Breukink and Donovan (2013) noted that while there have been some studies on men, there are few on women and even fewer on younger survivors. Much of what is known about sexual functioning in this population is based on extrapolations from other cancers or from the little evidence describing sexual functioning in older populations.

In women with anal or rectal cancer, impairment was seen across the spectrum of sexual functioning (e.g., desire, arousal, lubrication, orgasm, pain, satisfaction) (Philip et al., 2013). Some women in this study were not sexually active, but in those who were, a negative impact on emotional functioning was seen. The researchers posited that sexual activity may serve as a reminder of the disease experience and the distressing changes to physical functioning. In this study, body image was found to be strongly associated with sexual functioning.

Contraception

While it is increasingly recognized that attention must be paid to fertility and sexuality in young adults, other equally important issues, namely, contraception and safer sex, often are neglected. Some young adults will regain their ability to conceive or impregnate a partner after cancer; however, they may not be aware of this, instead assuming they are not fertile (Laurence, Gbolade, Morgan, & Glaser, 2004). Young adult cancer survivors have the same needs as their unaffected peers for high-quality education about safer sex and access to contraception. They are equally at risk for sexually transmitted infections (STIs) that may have more dire consequences because of survivors' compromised immunity, and the interruption to their lives from an unintended pregnancy may further complicate educational plans that have already been compromised by extended hospital stays or treatment regimens.

In a review of contraception for teenagers and young adults with cancer, Laurence et al. (2004) discussed the current contraceptive methods, including no method, withdrawal before ejaculation, and periodic abstinence. These are all associated with high risks of unintended pregnancy and do not protect against STIs. *Barrier methods* (the female condom and male condom) are available widely and do not require involvement of a healthcare provider. They protect against STIs and, if used correctly and consistently, are effective in preventing pregnancy. The male condom is relatively cheap, whereas the female condom is more expensive and more difficult to purchase because it is not as widely available, especially outside of urban centers. Condoms are also highly recommended for use while survivors are receiving chemotherapy because they protect partners from exposure to the metabolites of chemotherapy agents in body fluids. Male condoms are lubricated with a spermicidal jelly but should be used with extra lubrication (water- or silicone-based, never oil-based) to prevent breakage. Barrier methods require planning, and their use is often cited as interfering with spontaneity. Other barrier methods include the diaphragm and cervical cap. These are both female controlled and must be used with spermicidal jelly. They can be inserted before sexual intercourse and do not require the participation or even knowledge of the partner. They must be left in place for six to eight hours after intercourse. These methods require motivation as well as comfort with touching the genitalia for insertion and removal, and they have a fairly high failure rate, mostly because of inconsistent use and poor technique.

Hormonal methods include the oral contraceptive pill (containing estrogen and progestin), intravaginal ring, or patch (the intrauterine device, which contains progestin, will be discussed later in this section). The oral contraceptive pill, patch, or ring can be used by all young women except those with breast cancer. Efficacy is dependent on consistent use. The patch and ring need to be changed every month, whereas the pill needs to be taken daily. Complications from cancer treatment may affect the use of hormonal methods. For example, thrombocytopenia can cause excessive menstrual bleeding, and continuous use of the pill (without the week break in the 28-day pack of pills) may be helpful. Gastrointestinal side effects, such as vomiting, diarrhea, or mucositis, as well as prolonged use of antibiotics for febrile neutropenia, may affect absorption of the pill and lessen the effectiveness of this method to prevent pregnancy. Oral contraceptive pills should also be avoided in women after allogeneic bone marrow transplantation who require steroids and cyclosporins for prevention of graft-versus-host disease or rejection of the transplant. The progestin-only pill is an inferior oral contraceptive with a greater risk of failure than the combined estrogen-progestin pill. It is not recommended as first-line contraception for women with cancer.

The injectable contraceptive, depot medroxyprogesterone, is a long-acting hormonal method of contraception. The injection is given every 12 weeks and has a low failure rate. However, it is given as a deep intramuscular injection and is not suitable for those with a risk of thrombocytopenia or neutropenia because of the risk of hematoma formation or infection. Also, long-term use is associated with loss of bone density.

The intrauterine device (with one version containing progestin) is a well-established method of contraception. However, it is not recommended in young women who have not had a pregnancy. It also must be used with great caution in those with multiple sexual partners because it is associated with pelvic inflammatory disease in this population. It is contraindicated in women with a risk of neutropenia or thrombocytopenia.

The use of an emergency contraceptive immediately after unprotected intercourse or in the event of barrier method failure (condom slippage or breakage) is not contraindicated other than in women with breast cancer. Young adults with cancer should receive education about this method for use in emergencies only. Included in this education should be information about where to purchase the medication (it is available over the counter in some jurisdictions, pharmacist-controlled in others, and by prescription only in some) as well as the need for immediate action to prevent pregnancy.

None of these hormonal methods protect against STIs. This is a major concern for cancer survivors who may be immunocompromised and more susceptible to infection or whose health would be placed at risk by additional infection. Ideally, dual methods should be used when possible—an effective hormonal contraceptive with consistent condom use by the male partner.

How to Help the Young Adult With Cancer

Interventions

A limited number of interventions are available for sexual problems in men and women after cancer, and very few are directed at young adults. This may, in part, reflect the paucity of studies of young adults with cancer in general and a lack of attention to sexual issues across all age groups.

Stevenson and Elliott (2007) described sexual rehabilitation as maximizing physiologic capacity, adapting to residual limitations through the use of specialized therapies, and persistence in trying to succeed in rehabilitation with both the survivor and partner maintaining a positive outlook. Krychman and Millheiser (2013) addressed the topic of sexual rehabilitation medicine for women in their review. They described the goal of survivors' achieving a new normal in sexual functioning as opposed to returning to their previous level of functioning. They suggested a review of survivors' medication use with consideration given to finding alternatives to those agents that may be exacerbating sexual problems. For example, the selective serotonin reuptake inhibitors used to treat depression are known to cause sexual problems, and switching to another class or type of medication may help. They proposed that proper nutrition, avoidance of alcohol, and regular exercise also can help with sexual recovery. Various homework activities, such as sensate focus exercises, self-stimulation, erotic reading assignments, and relaxation techniques, may be helpful (Krychman & Millheiser, 2013).

In terms of pharmaceutical solutions, there are no U.S. Food and Drug Administration–approved medications for low desire or arousal in women. Local estrogen in pill, ring, or cream formulations is available for the treatment of vaginal atrophy, but its use in women with hormone-dependent cancers is controversial. Systemic hormone therapy can be prescribed for menopausal symptoms in women with cancers that are not hormone dependent (Krychman & Millheiser, 2013).

Nonhormonal vaginal moisturizers (e.g., Replens®) or vitamin E oil may provide some relief of daily discomfort. Lubricants should be used for sex play and vaginal penetration, and many different types and brands are available in drugstores, from online retailers, or in sex stores. Women should be aware of the risk of irritation from products that claim to be intensifying, warming, or cooling. Perfumes, dyes, flavors, and spermicides are all irritants, and careful reading of labels should be encouraged. Water-based lubricants are usually safe, but caution should be used because even these may contain irritants. Silicone-based lubricants should not be used with dilators, sex toys, diaphragms, or cervical caps.

Women who have received radiation to the pelvis as part of their treatment for gynecologic or colorectal cancer are encouraged to use dilators on a regular basis (or to have penetrative intercourse regularly) to prevent stenosis of the vagina; however, compliance with this is often low (Incrocci & Jensen, 2013). Women with gynecologic cancer can use local estrogen cream for relief of vaginal atrophy, which may improve the health of vaginal membranes.

Men who experience erectile difficulties after cancer treatment may respond to oral erectile aids such as sildenafil, tadalafil, or vardenafil. Achieving erections may boost libido in men who have lost sexual interest in response to challenges in achieving and maintaining erections. More invasive interventions, such as penile self-injection, may be required for men who do not respond to the oral agents. Erections are not purely a physical phenomenon, and some men may have a significant psychological component that will not respond to medication. Low libido in men after cancer treatment often is related to low testosterone levels. Correction of this with supplemental testosterone may be indicated in the absence of hormone-dependent cancers.

Hersch, Juraskova, Price, and Mullan (2009) reviewed psychosocial or psychological interventions to manage sexual problems after gynecologic cancer. They reported that counseling or cognitive-behavioral interventions did not improve self-esteem or body image. They found some very limited evidence for psychoeducational interventions specific to sexual functioning. Lori Brotto has pioneered a mindfulness-based cognitive behavioral intervention for women with gynecologic cancer. In one study (Brotto et al., 2008), women attended a three-session psychoeducational intervention that combined cognitive-behavioral therapy with education and mindfulness training. A significant improvement occurred in sexual desire, arousal, orgasm, satisfaction, and general well-being, and depression and distress decreased. The women in the study reported that the mindfulness part of the intervention was particularly helpful. The second study (Brotto et al., 2012) compared women with gynecologic cancer who attended three sessions of mindfulness-based cognitive-behavioral therapy with a wait-list control group. The women in the intervention group showed significant improvements in all sexual domains and, although a statistically significant improvement in distress did not occur, a trend was observed. Women in this group also reported increased perception of genital arousal in response to viewing an erotic movie.

A sexuality clinic (the SHARE clinic) developed by the nursing department of a hospital in Canada that provided education and supportive counseling to women with gynecologic cancer was shown to elicit high levels of satisfaction from the women who attended the clinic (Barbera et al., 2011).

The evaluation did not ask about improvements in symptom experience. A feasibility study of a 12-week Internet-based psychoeducational intervention showed that women will participate in this type of intervention. However, the study did not look at effectiveness or other treatment-related outcomes (Classen et al., 2013).

In a review of interventions for sexual problems after breast cancer (Taylor, Harley, Ziegler, Brown, & Velikova, 2011), only psychoeducational interventions that contained elements of sex therapy were found to be effective. These interventions were provided to survivors and their partners, survivors individually, or in groups. The educational component used skill-based training in the following areas: problem solving, communication, hypnosis, education, and specific sex therapy.

Canada, Schover, and Li (2007) reported on a pilot intervention to improve psychosexual development in adolescents and young adults with cancer. The intervention focused on education and support on topics such as sexual development and sexual functioning, body image, prevention of STIs, fertility, and contraception. The intervention showed positive results that were maintained through three months after the intervention. Knowledge about sexual issues improved, as did body image. Participants reported decreased anxiety about sexual and romantic relationships and overall distress.

Communication

Despite the prevalence of sexual difficulties for cancer survivors and the importance of sexuality in the lives of young adults, the issue is not addressed routinely by healthcare providers of all types, including physicians (Bober, Carter, & Falk, 2013; Park et al., 2009) and nurses (Olsson, Berglund, Larsson, & Athlin, 2012). Reasons for this include lack of knowledge, time constraints, embarrassment on the part of the provider, fear of causing offense to the patient, belief that the responsibility lies with another member of the healthcare team, and regarding this as unimportant (Julien, Thom, & Kline, 2010; Kotronoulas, Papadopoulou, & Patiraki, 2009).

Some healthcare providers are afraid that asking about sexual changes after treatment will result in the need for an extended counseling session that they are not equipped to provide, so they avoid asking the question. Others say that they do not know what to ask or how to introduce the topic. Survivors and their partners may interpret this lack of inquiry as indicating that the topic is not important or even taboo. However, assessment of sexuality is recognized as an important part of comprehensive and holistic care of people with cancer and, as such, should be addressed in a systematic way with all patients. Studies have shown that healthcare providers in general neglect sexuality assessment. Park et al. (2009) reported that 46% of internists were likely to initiate a conversation about sexual dysfunction with cancer survivors, while 62% rarely or never talked about the topic. A study of gynecologic oncologists found that less than 50% took a sexual history from their patients and that 80% reported not having enough time to do this, despite acknowledged sexual problems in this population (Wiggins, Wood, Granai, & Dizon, 2007).

What are survivors' experiences related to communication with health-care providers? In a study of survivors with different kinds of cancer with participants of all ages, 74% of those in the study felt that discussions with oncology care providers about sexual issues were important, yet most did not have any discussion. Only 29% of breast and 39% of colorectal cancer survivors had received information about sexuality from their oncology care providers (Flynn et al., 2012). It is important to talk about these issues with patients, as they want and need to know how to deal with sexual side effects.

Althof and Parish (2013) suggested that in general, sexual health interviewing skills encompass screening, assessment, open-ended questions, empathetic delineation, and counseling. Screening involves general questions about sexual functioning to create a baseline before treatment against which future sexual functioning may be compared (e.g., "Tell me about your last sexual encounter. Did you experience any difficulties?" "Many young women who have been treated for cancer have problems with sexuality; how about you?") Assessment of any sexual problems identified involves a thorough evaluation of the problem including when it happens, triggers, intensity, whether it is lifelong or newly acquired, whether the onset was gradual or sudden, what other factors may be contributing to it, and what level of distress or bother the problem is causing. Open-ended questions should be used to encourage a full narrative response to questions. Prompts such as "Tell me more" and "What is the most distressing thing about this for you?" allow for full descriptions that are not elicited with a closed-ended approach. *Empathetic delineation* is a therapeutic technique that encourages patients to begin solving their problems by linking the distress they experience to motivation to get help (Althof & Parish, 2013). Normalizing sexual problems as a consequence of cancer treatment, validating the emotional response to the problem, and reframing the sexual problem as a priority that needs to be dealt with are aspects of empathetic delineation. Finally, Althof and Parish suggested that while patients may be reluctant to seek or accept counseling, using patient-centered techniques such as motivational interviewing can encourage them to engage in counseling to solve their problems.

A number of specific assessment tools exist that can be used to guide the conversation about sexuality and the sexual side effects of treatment. A simple question such as "How has your sexuality been affected by your cancer or its treatment?" may be enough to elicit a detailed response from the survivor. Situating the question in the context of the relationship (e.g., "How has your relationship with your partner/girlfriend/boyfriend been affected by the cancer?") may make asking the question easier, although a prompt about the specific sexual changes may still be necessary.

The following assessment frameworks will be helpful in initiating conversations about changes to sexuality during and after cancer.

The **PLISSIT model** (Anon, 1974) is a well-known assessment tool that has been used extensively in sexual health assessment and counseling. This four-part model starts with *permission*, where the healthcare provider makes an opening statement suggesting to the patients/survivors that it is acceptable to ask questions about sexuality, that what they are going through is common or expected, or that it is normal to feel the way they are feeling. The next stage, *limited information*, allows the healthcare provider to provide basic information in response to a question or in validation of patients' experiences. This information is purposively not in-depth but rather represents enough to answer the question without overwhelming patients. The next level, *specific suggestion*, requires the healthcare provider to make suggestions to resolve the sexual problems that patients are experiencing and requires a deeper level of knowledge and understanding on the part of the healthcare provider. The last level, *intensive therapy*, is usually beyond the scope of the frontline healthcare provider and requires referral to specialized sexual counseling or therapy.

Taylor and Davis (2007) proposed a modification to the PLISSIT model. They suggested that the model is often used in a way that is limited. For example, they stated that the permission stage is often ignored and patients are provided with written information about their condition and sexual functioning, and that by not giving permission, the healthcare provider implies that sexuality is not something to be talked about. They also suggested that many healthcare providers give permission once in an interaction with patients, and if patients do not ask a question or voice a concern, providers assume there are no problems and never ask again. In response to these criticisms, Taylor and Davis suggested an extended approach, Ex-PLISSIT.

The **Ex-PLISSIT model** suggests that permission is the core of this process and should be used at each level of the model and repeated at each interaction with patients. For example, beyond the initial permission giving, practitioners should give permission to patients before offering limited information. A statement such as "Many men experience low libido after stem cell transplantation. Is this something you have experienced?" is an example of limited information. This question focuses on a side effect of transplantation that is beyond the basic permission-giving level. For the specific suggestion level, permission giving may include a statement such as "Some men find that their libido doesn't return spontaneously. Would you like to talk about treatment that might help with this?" Permission giving here requires the patient to agree to learn something more about dealing with the consequences of treatment and consideration of further interventions to alleviate the problem.

This repeated permission giving allows patients to divulge information about their own circumstances as they are comfortable doing so and provides opportunities for providers to educate patients about the specifics of their situation, rather than in a more generalized fashion. This helps to prevent providers from making assumptions about patients, for example, talking to a woman about positions for sexual intercourse when the woman does not participate in this activity because she is not partnered at the time.

In addition, Taylor and Davis (2007) suggested that rather than proceed through the three levels before referring for intensive therapy, this can be done at any stage. Practitioners must be aware of their own strengths and limitations as well as their scope of practice and not go beyond those. And this referral is not only for intensive sex therapy; the specialist may provide care in other spheres such as sexual medicine, gynecology, urology, etc.

Finally, the process of reflection and review is part of the Ex-PLISSIT model whereby practitioners are challenged to constantly reflect on what they have been told and then review the information given to and received from patients. This reflection on the part of the practitioner encourages questioning of one's own attitudes and beliefs and helps to dispel assumptions. The review with the patient allows for consideration of broader consequences. For example, after suggesting further testing and treatment of low libido, the practitioner might ask about what the man's partner/spouse thinks about the situation. A review should also take place at the start of future appointments wherein patients are asked what they learned from the educational material provided at the last appointment or whether a suggestion made at the time was acted upon and what the result was.

Another framework, the **5 A's**, was originally developed for tobacco cessation, but it has application for sexual health or dysfunction assessment and is already familiar to many healthcare providers (Bober et al., 2013).

1. **Ask** about sexual health. A simple question such as those offered earlier in the chapter initiates the conversation.
2. **Advise** patients that they are not alone or unique in experiencing the problem. This validation is often enough to allay their fears.
3. **Assess** any problems or issues raised in response to the question. This can be done by further questioning about frequency and severity of the symptom or symptoms, as well as the associated distress or burden.
4. **Assist** patients by providing them with resources that can help, including reading material, websites, and information sheets. Referrals to a sexual medicine provider or counselor/therapist may be necessary or preferred by patients.
5. **Arrange** follow-up and ask at all subsequent appointments about resolution or management of the problem or problems identified. This will

facilitate timely referral if the problem persists or worsens and indicates to patients that this is an important issue.

This model may be particularly useful in the primary care setting, where it has been used and is well understood in the context of smoking cessation. The framework is easy to remember and follows a stepwise approach that is intuitive to many healthcare providers. However, it does not appear to have been tested and validated for this purpose.

The **BETTER model** (Mick, Hughes, & Cohen, 2003) was developed for use by oncology nurses who want to address sexuality with their patients. It is prescriptive in what nurses must address with patients, including side effects of treatment and the rationale for asking (quality of life). The stages of the BETTER model are

- **B**ring up the topic.
- **E**xplain you are concerned with quality-of-life issues, including sexuality.
- **T**ell patients that resources will be found to answer their questions or concerns.
- **T**iming may not seem appropriate now, but they can ask for information or help at any time.
- **E**ducate patients about the side effects of their cancer treatment.
- **R**ecord the interaction in the medical record.

Other models of sexuality assessment are available that are more biomedical in their approach, such as the **ALARM model** (Andersen, 1990). This model is based on the Masters and Johnson human sexual response cycle. Questions are asked in the following five areas.

- **A**ctivity: Frequency of current sexual activities (intercourse, kissing, masturbation)
- **L**ibido/desire: Desire for sexual activity and interest in initiating or responding to partner
- **A**rousal and orgasm: Occurrence of erection/lubrication and orgasm accompanied with feelings of sexual excitement
- **R**esolution: Feelings of release of tension following sexual activity and satisfaction with current sexual life
- **M**edical history: Current age, medical status, and psychiatric and substance abuse history

Contraceptive and Safer Sex Counseling

Healthcare providers often assume that young adults have the knowledge and experience to protect themselves against an unwanted pregnancy or STIs. Some may feel that it is the exclusive role of the parents and perhaps even the school system to do this. But parents and schools may not provide this education to young people and certainly not in the context of cancer treatment and survivorship. Healthcare providers also may have their own beliefs and attitudes about sex before marriage or the "acceptable" age to begin sexual activity and subsequently do not ask or educate young patients about this topic. This is potentially dangerous for younger patients who may not think about the risks associated with chemotherapy or radiation and pregnancy, and not providing them with the information to protect their partners and themselves is neglectful and could be regarded as a failure to protect. Healthcare providers also may think that providing written information to young adults as they do for older adults is sufficient. But the written materials given to older adults do not address the unique needs of this population, who may not read anything given to them in the first place.

It is essential to provide young adults with accurate information about preventing pregnancy during treatment and for some time post-treatment for certain cancers. It is always important to provide anticipatory guidance about preventing STIs, as acquiring one will complicate treatment, recovery, and the rest of their lives.

Websites such as Go Ask Alice! (http://goaskalice.columbia.edu) and My Beautiful Sex Life (www.guidetogettingiton.com) provide excellent evidence-based information for young adults and healthcare providers.

It is also important to recognize that young adults may be embarrassed to speak to older healthcare providers. If possible, referral to a specialized sexuality professional such as a sexuality counselor or therapist may be highly beneficial and may lessen feelings of embarrassment. But it may be challenging to find professionals to refer to. The American Association of Sexuality Educators, Counselors, and Therapists (www.aasect.org) has a list of certified practitioners who may be able to provide consultation for both patients and staff.

Conclusion

Talking about sex is difficult for many healthcare providers, and the evidence suggests that this area of oncology care is frequently ignored or neglected. Healthcare providers have a duty to provide anticipatory guidance and education to young adults who, by being sexual, are achieving one of their important developmental milestones, despite the challenges of their illness. By maintaining silence about this topic, oncology professionals ultimately reinforce a taboo suggesting that sex is not healthy. This, in turn, maintains the isolation of young adults who are only doing (or wanting to do) what comes naturally and is something that many adults enjoy and celebrate, particularly in the aftermath of cancer. It makes people feel alive and "normal" again and is a sentinel aspect of survivorship and should be something that all cancer survivors can enjoy.

References

Abbott-Anderson, K., & Kwekkeboom, K.L. (2012). A systematic review of sexual concerns reported by gynecologic cancer survivors. *Gynecologic Oncology, 124,* 477–489. doi:10.1016/j.ygyno.2011.11.030

Althof, S.E., & Parish, S.J. (2013). Clinical interviewing techniques and sexuality questionnaires for male and female cancer patients. *Journal of Sexual Medicine, 10*(Suppl. 1), 35–42. doi:10.1111/jsm.12035

Andersen, B.L. (1990). How cancer affects sexual functioning. *Oncology, 4*(6), 81–94.

Andersen, B.L. (2009). In sickness and in health: Maintaining intimacy after breast cancer recurrence. *Cancer Journal, 15,* 70–73. doi:10.1097/PPO.0b013e318198c742

Anon, J.S. (1974). *The behavioral treatment of sexual problems.* Honolulu, HI: Enabling Systems.

Arden-Close, E., Eiser, C., & Pacey, A. (2011). Sexual functioning in male survivors of lymphoma: A systematic review. *Journal of Sexual Medicine, 8,* 1833–1840. doi:10.1111/j.1743-6109.2011.02209.x

Bakewell, R.T., & Volker, D.L. (2005). Sexual dysfunction related to the treatment of young women with breast cancer. *Clinical Journal of Oncology Nursing, 9,* 697–702. doi:10.1188/05.CJON.697-702

Barbera, L., Fitch, M., Adams, L., Doyle, C., DasGupta, T., & Blake, J. (2011). Improving care for women after gynecological cancer: The development of a sexuality clinic. *Menopause, 18,* 1327–1333. doi:10.1097/gme.0b013e31821f598c

Basson, R. (2005). Women's sexual dysfunction: Revised and expanded definitions. *Canadian Medical Association Journal, 172,* 1327–1333. doi:10.1503/cmaj.1020174

Beesley, H., Ullmer, H., Holcombe, C., & Salmon, P. (2012). How patients evaluate breast reconstruction after mastectomy, and why their evaluation often differs from that of their clinicians. *Journal of Plastic, Reconstructive and Aesthetic Surgery, 65,* 1064–1071. doi:10.1016/j.bjps.2012.03.005

Behringer, K., Müller, H., Görgen, H., Flechtner, H.-H., Brillant, C., Halbsguth, T.V., ... Borchmann, P. (2013). Sexual quality of life in Hodgkin lymphoma: A longitudinal analysis by the German Hodgkin Study Group. *British Journal of Cancer,* 49–57. doi:10.1038/bjc.2012.550

Bober, S.L., Carter, J., & Falk, S. (2013). Addressing female sexual function after cancer by internists and primary care providers. *Journal of Sexual Medicine, 10*(Suppl. 1), 112–119. doi:10.1111/jsm.12027

Boquiren, V.M., Esplen, M.J., Wong, J., Toner, B., & Warner, E. (2013). Exploring the influence of gender-role socialization and objectified body consciousness on body image disturbance in breast cancer survivors. *Psycho-Oncology.* Advance online publication. doi:10.1002/pon.3271

Brédart, A., Dolbeault, S., Savignoni, A., Besancenet, C., This, P., Giami, A., ... Copel, L. (2011). Prevalence and associated factors of sexual problems after early-stage breast cancer treatment: Results of a French exploratory survey. *Psycho-Oncology, 20,* 841–850. doi:10.1002/pon.1789

Breukink, S.O., & Donovan, K.A. (2013). Physical and psychological effects of treatment on sexual functioning in colorectal cancer survivors. *Journal of Sexual Medicine, 10*(Suppl. 1), 74–83. doi:10.1111/jsm.12037

Brotto, L.A., Erskine, Y., Carey, M., Ehlen, T., Finlayson, S., Heywood, M., ... Miller, D. (2012). A brief mindfulness-based cognitive behavioral intervention improves sexual functioning versus wait-list control in women treated for gynecologic cancer. *Gynecologic Oncology, 125,* 320–325. doi:10.1016/j.ygyno.2012.01.035

Brotto, L.A., Heiman, J.R., Goff, B., Greer, B., Lentz, G.M., Swisher, E., ... Van Blaricom, A. (2008). A psychoeducational intervention for sexual dysfunction in women with gynecologic cancer. *Archives of Sexual Behavior, 37,* 317–329. doi:10.1007/s10508-007-9196-x

Campos, S.M., Berlin, S., Matulonis, U.A., Muto, M.G., Pereira, L., Mosquera, M.M., & Horowitz, N. (2012). Young women diagnosed with early-stage ovarian cancer or borderline malignancy of the ovary: A focus on fertility and sexual function. *Journal of Psychosocial Oncology, 30,* 387–401. doi:10.1080/07347332.2012.684854

Canada, A., Schover, L., & Li, Y. (2007). A pilot intervention to enhance psychosexual development in adolescents and young adults with cancer. *Pediatric Blood and Cancer, 49,* 824–828. doi:10.1002/pbc.21130

Carpenter, K.M., Andersen, B.L., Fowler, J.M., & Maxwell, G.L. (2009). Sexual self schema as a moderator of sexual and psychological outcomes for gynecologic cancer survivors. *Archives of Sexual Behavior, 38,* 828–841. doi:10.1007/s10508-008-9349-6

Carpentier, M.Y., Fortenberry, J.D., Ott, M.A., Brames, M.J., & Einhorn, L.H. (2011). Perceptions of masculinity and self-image in adolescent and young adult testicular cancer survivors: Implications for romantic and sexual relationships. *Psycho-Oncology, 20,* 738–745. doi:10.1002/pon.1772

Carter, J., Stabile, C., Gunn, A., & Sonoda, Y. (2013). The physical consequences of gynecologic cancer surgery and their impact on sexual, emotional, and quality of life issues. *Journal of Sexual Medicine, 10*(Suppl. 1), 21–34. doi:10.1111/jsm.12002

Classen, C.C., Chivers, M.L., Urowitz, S., Barbera, L., Wiljer, D., O'Rinn, S., & Ferguson, S.E. (2013). Psychosexual distress in women with gynecologic cancer: A feasibility study of an online support group. *Psycho-Oncology, 22,* 930–935. doi:10.1002/pon.3058

Donovan, K.A., Thompson, L.M., & Hoffe, S.E. (2010). Sexual function in colorectal cancer survivors. *Cancer Control, 17,* 44–51.

Eeltink, C.M., Incrocci, L., Witte, B.I., Meurs, S., Visser, O., Huijgens, P., & Verdonck-de Leeuw, I.M. (2013). Fertility and sexual function in female Hodgkin lymphoma survivors of reproductive age. *Journal of Clinical Nursing, 22,* 3513–3521. doi:10.1111/jocn.12354

Fang, S.-Y., Shu, B.-C., & Chang, Y.-J. (2013). The effect of breast reconstruction surgery on body image among women after mastectomy: A meta-analysis. *Breast Cancer Research and Treatment, 137,* 13–21. doi:10.1007/s10549-012-2349-1

Flynn, K.E., Reese, J.B., Jeffery, D.D., Abernethy, A.P., Lin, L., Shelby, R.A., ... Weinfurt, K.P. (2012). Patient experiences with communication about sex during and after treatment for cancer. *Psycho-Oncology, 21,* 594–601. doi:10.1002/pon.1947

Frumovitz, M., Sun, C.C., Schover, L.R., Munsell, M.F., Jhingran, A., Wharton, J.T., ... Bodurka, D.C. (2005). Quality of life and sexual functioning in cervical cancer survivors. *Journal of Clinical Oncology, 23,* 7428–7436. doi:10.1200/JCO.2004.00.3996

Gershenson, D.M., Miller, A.M., Champion, V.L., Monahan, P.O., Zhao, Q., Cella, D., & Williams, S.D. (2007). Reproductive and sexual function after platinum-based chemotherapy in long-term ovarian germ cell tumor survivors: A Gynecologic Oncology Group study. *Journal of Clinical Oncology, 25,* 2792–2797. doi:10.1200/JCO.2006.08.4590

Greimel, E.R., Winter, R., Kapp, K.S., & Haas, J. (2009). Quality of life and sexual functioning after cervical cancer treatment: A long-term follow-up study. *Psycho-Oncology, 18,* 476–482. doi:10.1002/pon.1426

Hersch, J., Juraskova, I., Price, M., & Mullan, B. (2009). Psychosocial interventions and quality of life in gynaecological cancer patients: A systematic review. *Psycho-Oncology, 18,* 795–810. doi:10.1002/pon.1443

Incrocci, L., & Jensen, P.T. (2013). Pelvic radiotherapy and sexual function in men and women. *Journal of Sexual Medicine, 10*(Suppl. 1), 53–64. doi:10.1111/jsm.12010

Jankowska, M. (2013). Sexual functioning in young women in the context of breast cancer treatment. *Reports of Practical Oncology and Radiotherapy, 18,* 193–200. doi:10.1016/j.rpor.2013.04.032

Julien, J.O., Thom, B., & Kline, N.E. (2010). Identification of barriers to sexual health assessment in oncology nursing practice [Online exclusive]. *Oncology Nursing Forum, 37,* E186–E190. doi:10.1188/10.ONF.E186-E190

Juraskova, I., Butow, P., Bonner, C., Robertson, R., & Sharpe, L. (2013). Sexual adjustment following early stage cervical and endometrial cancer: Prospective controlled multi-centre study. *Psycho-Oncology, 22,* 153–159. doi:10.1002/pon.2066

Kaplan, H.S. (1979). *Disorders of sexual desire and other new concepts and techniques in sex therapy.* New York, NY: Simon & Schuster.

Kelly, D. (2013). Developing age appropriate psychosexual support for adolescent cancer survivors: A discussion paper. *Journal of Sexual Medicine, 10*(Suppl. 1), 133–138. doi:10.1111/jsm.12048

Kim, C., McGlynn, K.A., McCorkle, R., Li, Y., Erickson, R.L., Ma, S., ... Zhang, Y. (2012). Sexual functioning among testicular cancer survivors: A case-control study in the U.S. *Journal of Psychosomatic Research, 73,* 68–73. doi:10.1016/j.jpsychores.2012.02.011

Kotronoulas, G., Papadopoulou, C., & Patiraki, E. (2009). Nurses' knowledge, attitudes, and practices regarding provision of sexual health care in patients with cancer: Critical review of the evidence. *Supportive Care in Cancer, 17,* 479–501. doi:10.1007/s00520-008-0563-5

Krychman, M., & Millheiser, L.S. (2013). Sexual health issues in women with cancer. *Journal of Sexual Medicine, 10*(Suppl. 1), 5–15. doi:10.1111/jsm.12034

Laurence, V., Gbolade, B.A., Morgan, S.J., & Glaser, A. (2004). Contraception for teenagers and young adults with cancer. *European Journal of Cancer, 40,* 2705–2716. doi:10.1016/j.ejca.2004.09.003

Markopoulos, C., Tsaroucha, A.K., Kouskos, E., Mantas, D., Antonopoulou, Z., & Karvelis, S. (2009). Impact of breast cancer surgery on the self-esteem and sexual life of female patients. *Journal of International Medical Research, 37,* 182–188. doi:10.1177/147323000903700122

Masters, W.H., & Johnson, V.E. (1966). *Human sexual response.* Boston, MA: Little, Brown.

Mick, J., Hughes, M., & Cohen, M.Z. (2003). Sexuality and cancer: How oncology nurses can address it BETTER (Abstract No. 180). *Oncology Nursing Forum, 30*(Suppl.), 152–153.

Morgan, S., Davies, S., Palmer, S., & Plaster, M. (2010). Sex, drugs, and rock 'n' roll: Caring for adolescents and young adults with cancer. *Journal of Clinical Oncology, 28,* 4825–4830. doi:10.1200/JCO.2009.22.5474

Olsson, C., Berglund, A.L., Larsson, M., & Athlin, E. (2012). Patient's sexuality—A neglected area of cancer nursing? *European Journal of Oncology Nursing, 16,* 426–431. doi:10.1016/j.ejon.2011.10.003

Park, E.R., Bober, S.L., Campbell, E.G., Recklitis, C.J., Kutner, J.S., & Diller, L. (2009). General internist communication about sexual function with cancer survivors. *Journal of General Internal Medicine, 24*(Suppl. 2), S407–S411. doi:10.1007/s11606-009-1026-5

Philip, E.J., Nelson, C., Temple, L., Carter, J., Schover, L., Jennings, S., ... DuHamel, K. (2013). Psychological correlates of sexual dysfunction in female rectal and anal cancer survivors: Analysis of baseline intervention data. *Journal of Sexual Medicine, 10,* 2539–2548. doi:10.1111/jsm.12152

Ratner, E.S., Foran, K.A., Schwartz, P.E., & Minkin, M.J. (2010). Sexuality and intimacy after gynecological cancer. *Maturitas, 66,* 23–26. doi:10.1016/j.maturitas.2010.01.015

Recklitis, C.J., Varela, V.S., Ng, A., Mauch, P., & Bober, S. (2010). Sexual functioning in long-term survivors of Hodgkin's lymphoma. *Psycho-Oncology, 19,* 1229–1233. doi:10.1002/pon.1679

Rosenberg, S.M., Tamimi, R.M., Gelber, S., Ruddy, K.J., Bober, S.L., Kereakoglow, S., ... Partridge, A.H. (2014). Treatment-related amenorrhea and sexual functioning in young breast cancer survivors. *Cancer, 120,* 2264–2271. doi:10.1002/cncr.28738

Rosenberg, S.M., Tamimi, R.M., Gelber, S., Ruddy, K.J., Kereakoglow, S., Borges, V.F., ... Partridge, A.H. (2012). Body image in recently diagnosed young women with early breast cancer. *Psycho-Oncology, 22,* 1849–1855. doi:10.1002/pon.3221

Schover, L.R. (2014). Premature ovarian failure is a major risk factor for cancer-related sexual dysfunction. *Cancer, 120,* 2230–2232. doi:10.1002/cncr.28735

Sekse, R.J.T., Gjengedal, E., & Råheim, M. (2013). Living in a changed female body after gynecological cancer. *Health Care for Women International, 34,* 14–33. doi:10.1080/07399332.2011.645965

Stevenson, R.W.D., & Elliott, S.L. (2007). Sexuality and illness. In S.R. Leiblum (Ed.), *Principles and practice of sex therapy* (4th ed., pp. 313–349). New York, NY: Guilford Press.

Taylor, B., & Davis, S. (2007). The extended PLISSIT model for addressing the sexual wellbeing of individuals with an acquired disability or chronic illness. *Sexuality and Disability, 25,* 135–139. doi:10.1007/s11195-007-9044-x

Taylor, S., Harley, C., Ziegler, L., Brown, J., & Velikova, G. (2011). Interventions for sexual problems following treatment for breast cancer: A systematic review. *Breast Cancer Research and Treatment, 130,* 711–724. doi:10.1007/s10549-011-1722-9

Ussher, J., Perz, J., & Gilbert, E. (2012). Changes to sexual well-being and intimacy after breast cancer. *Cancer Nursing, 35,* 456–465. doi:10.1097/NCC.0b013e3182395401

Wiggins, D.L., Wood, R., Granai, C.O., & Dizon, D.S. (2007). Sex, intimacy, and the gynecologic oncologist. *Journal of Psychosocial Oncology, 25,* 61–70. doi:10.1300/J077v25n04_04

CHAPTER 6
Fertility Challenges

Introduction

Being able to have children is an important dream for many people, including cancer survivors. Starting a family is an important developmental milestone and one that is threatened by cancer and its treatments. However, having had cancer is not the end of this dream for all cancer survivors—modern reproductive technology has made the possibility of having a child or children a reality for some survivors.

The effects of cancer treatment on fertility are dependent on many factors, including the kind of cancer, the type of treatment, the intensity or dose of the treatment, and the age of patients at the time of treatment. Preserving or protecting future fertility is also dependent on multiple factors, including whether this is discussed by healthcare providers with patients at an appropriate time, what techniques are available at the time of treatment, whether patients have a partner, whether they already have one or more children at the time, their economic and insurance status, and their access to fertility specialists. This chapter will describe the basics of male and female reproductive capacity, the impact of the various cancer treatments on fertility, fertility preservation methods, how people make decisions about preserving fertility, and the effects of altered fertility on cancer survivors.

Male Reproduction

Male fertility is dependent on two major factors. First, the testicles are under the influence of two hormones, follicle-stimulating hormone (FSH) and luteinizing hormone (LH), that control the production of the male sex hormone, testosterone. Second, testosterone acts on the testes in conjunction with FSH to promote spermatogenesis (Wallace,

2011). Postpubertal boys and men produce sperm continuously throughout life.

Surgery, radiation, and chemotherapy can affect sperm production. The effects of targeted therapy and immunotherapy are not well documented at the present time.

Impact of Surgery

The cancer in young men most likely to require surgical management is testicular cancer. Orchiectomy (surgical removal of the affected testicle) is the standard treatment, as it removes the tumor but also allows for histologic and pathologic staging and subsequent adjuvant treatment planning (Viatori, 2012). Loss of one testicle does not necessarily affect fertility. However, retroperitoneal lymph node dissection can affect ejaculation, which is necessary for natural conception (Viatori, 2012). Unilateral rather than bilateral nerve-sparing lymph node dissection is a technique that protects the nerves related to ejaculation, and this is the preferred approach when possible. Hypogonadism is common in men prior to diagnosis and is associated with subfertility (Gospodarowicz, 2008). The impact of orchiectomy on body image and sexuality is discussed in Chapter 5.

Impact of Chemotherapy

The testicles are highly sensitive to chemotherapy, especially alkylating agents. Lowered sperm count (oligospermia) or absent sperm (azoospermia) often results from these agents, which may be permanent changes despite normal testosterone levels (Wallace, 2011). There is frequently no choice in which chemotherapy agents are used; therefore, opting for treatment that is less toxic to spermatogenesis is usually not possible. Sperm banking is an important fertility preservation method and will be discussed in detail later in this chapter.

Impact of Radiation Therapy

Low doses of radiation therapy to the testicles can impair the production of sperm, and with higher doses, this may be permanent. The amount of radiation that men receive as part of the conditioning for bone marrow or stem cell transplantation will also affect sperm production. However, the high-dose chemotherapy used in preparation for transplantation also has an effect, so the exact contribution of the radiation to altered sperm production is difficult to assess (Wallace, 2011). When possible, the testes should be shielded during radiation treatment to minimize damage to spermatogenesis.

Female Reproduction

Baby girls are born with millions of ovarian follicles. Every month, under the influence of FSH and LH, one or more ovarian follicles mature, producing one or more ova (eggs). If the ovum (egg) is not fertilized, it is lost during menses. The number of ovarian follicles, and ova, declines over the life span of the woman, and by menopause only about 1,000 remain. As a woman ages, her ability to conceive declines as well; this is due to factors including age, smoking, obesity, and stress (Wallace, 2011). A woman's ability to bear children is thus, in part, dependent on healthy ovaries, uterine tubes, uterus, and cervix, all of which may be targets of cancer.

Impact of Surgery

Historically, gynecologic cancers have been treated with radical surgery that effectively removes any chance of the woman conceiving or carrying a fetus. Gynecologic cancer was treated with complete removal of the cervix, uterus, and ovaries.

Today, increased attention is being paid to fertility-preserving treatment where appropriate, depending on the grade and stage of disease. These more conservative treatments are available to only a select group of patients and include cervical tissue–sparing procedures for cervical cancer (conization or trachelectomy); hormone therapy alone for low-grade endometrial cancer followed by careful surveillance; and preservation of most of the unaffected contralateral ovary when possible for young women with early, localized ovarian cancer with low-risk pathology or for women with tumors of low malignant potential (Kesic, 2008).

Impact of Chemotherapy

As with men, the alkylating agents have the most profound effect on fertility for women with cancer. Damage to the ovaries is drug and dose dependent; however, the older the woman, the greater the risk that chemotherapy even at low doses will lead to ovarian failure. Chemotherapy in a young girl before puberty is likely to result in damage to ovarian follicles and subsequent risk to future fertility. Even if their periods resume after chemotherapy, young women are likely to experience premature menopause (Wallace, 2011).

The highest risk for infertility comes from stem cell transplantation with cyclophosphamide and total body irradiation. Intermediate risk to fertility results from adjuvant chemotherapy for breast cancer in women ages 30–39 including combinations of cyclophosphamide, methotrexate, fluorouracil, doxorubicin, and epirubicin. Lower risk to fertility is posed by regimens containing these drugs but in shorter cycles or for women under the age of 30. Very low risk is posed by methotrexate, fluorouracil, vincristine, bleomycin, or dactinomycin as single agents. The effects on fertility of the taxanes, oxaliplatin, irinotecan, monoclonal antibodies, and tyrosine kinase inhibitors are not yet known (Salama et al., 2013).

Impact of Radiation Therapy

Radiation to the pelvis or abdomen, including total body irradiation before bone marrow or stem cell transplantation, may adversely affect the blood vessels and muscles of the uterus. Uterine growth and elasticity are impacted, and this usually results in an inability to carry a pregnancy or to carry it to term. This is dose and age dependent, with higher doses resulting in greater damage. If the ovaries lie in the radiation field, they will also be affected (Wallace, 2011).

Fertility Preservation

The American Society of Clinical Oncology (ASCO) updated its guidelines on fertility preservation in 2013 (Loren et al., 2013). The guidelines state that all oncology care providers have a responsibility to discuss fertility preservation with patients of reproductive age, as well as with the parents or guardians of children and adolescents when treatment poses a risk to future fertility. The National Comprehensive Cancer Network® guidelines recommend that fertility preservation should be a key part in the treatment of adolescent and young adult patients whose fertility may be threatened by cancer (National Comprehensive Cancer Network, 2014).

The following section will discuss the latest evidence for fertility preservation techniques with the caveat that this is a rapidly changing field.

Preserving Male Fertility

Options for fertility preservation in men include sperm banking, testicular sperm extraction or aspiration, electroejaculation for sperm banking, and testicular tissue banking (Johnson & Kroon, 2013). Shielding the testes during radiation is also a method of fertility preservation. It does not provide assurance of future fertility but may mitigate damage, especially in young children who cannot bank sperm.

Sperm banking (cryopreservation) is the most established fertility preservation method. It does not require equipment or medical procedures. However, for younger men, especially young adolescents, it can be embarrassing, especially if discussed in front of parents or guardians or if they are involved in taking the young man to a fertility clinic. Mail-in kits are available so that it can be done at home, which alleviates some of the embarrassment. Banking sperm involves masturbation, and the recommendation is that the man produces two to three samples, with 48 hours between samples to maximize sperm counts. This is not always possible if treatment needs to start immediately. Because in vitro fertilization of a female partner now is usually done with intracytoplasmic sperm injection (ICSI), in which a single sperm is used to fertilize an ovum, large volume or multiple specimens typically are not necessary (Kenney et al., 2012). For men who were not able to bank sperm before treatment, waiting until 12 months after completion of treatment and then attempting to bank sperm may be possible (Katz, Kolon, Feldman, & Mulhall, 2013). Semen analysis needs to be performed to check whether men have viable sperm, but sperm banking would protect their hopes for future fertility in case of recurrence of the cancer.

Despite the relative simplicity and low risk of this method of fertility preservation, not all men offered sperm cryopreservation will follow through and bank sperm, and many of those who do will not use the banked sperm in the future. A recent study from Canada reported that 93% of men did not use their samples and 33% decided to destroy their samples after completion of cancer treatment. Ultimately, only 7% of men used their samples. Of the men who requested destruction of their samples, 32% reported that they had fathered a child spontaneously or completed their family (Olatunbosun & Zhu, 2012). Success rates with using cryopreserved sperm vary; in one study, pregnancies occurred in 36.4% of couples after intrauterine insemination and in 50% using in vitro fertilization or ICSI (Neal et al., 2007).

If the man cannot produce a semen sample by masturbation, sperm extraction or electroejaculation can be used. However, these procedures have to be performed under general anesthesia, and in some cases, the risks posed by this outweigh the potential benefits of sperm banking. Data are limited on experience with this method of procuring sperm, but theoretically the sperm should be able to be cryopreserved in the usual manner. One study reported success with both electroejaculation and testicular sperm extraction (Berookhim & Mulhall, 2014).

Testicular tissue cryopreservation (with the intent of reimplanting it after the cancer is treated) also is invasive and, at the time of writing, still highly experimental. Implanting tissue also raises the risk of reintroducing cancer cells into the body after treatment (Ruddy & Partridge, 2012).

Preserving Female Fertility

Preserving fertility in women is more complex than for men, with limited established techniques but promising experimental options. Established methods include embryo cryopreservation and, more recently, oocyte cryopreservation. Shielding of the ovaries or transposition of the ovaries out of the radiation field during therapy has been done for many years, and now intensity-modulated radiation therapy is also helpful in avoiding damage to the ovaries when possible. Experimental techniques include freezing ovarian tissue from prepubertal girls and ovarian suppression (Johnson & Kroon, 2013) (see Table 6-1).

Table 6-1. Options for Fertility Preservation for Women		
Technique	**Advantages**	**Disadvantages**
Embryo banking	Established technique Predictable success rates	Requires male gamete Time required for ovarian stimulation Potential for ethical issues with embryo disposition
Oocyte banking	Greater reproductive flexibility Improving efficacy	Experimental procedure Time required for ovarian stimulation
In vitro maturation of oocytes	Greater reproductive flexibility Avoids ovarian stimulation	Inferior oocyte yield compared to embryo/oocyte banking Similar time required for procedure as for embryo/oocyte banking
Ovarian tissue cryopreservation	Restoration of hormonal function Potential for future pregnancy without need for ART Option for prepubertal girls	Experimental procedure Unproven success rates Risk of reseeding tumor from micrometastases in ovarian tissue
Gonadal suppression with GnRH agonists	No surgical procedure Preserves hormonal function and fertility	Uncertain efficacy; mixed results from RCTs
Ovarian transposition	Decreases risk of ovarian failure from irradiation	Utility limited to patient with pelvic radiation Requires surgical procedure Lateral transposition may require IVF/ART if fallopian tube transected

ART—assisted reproductive techniques; GnRH—gonadotropin-releasing hormone; IVF—in vitro fertilization; RCT—randomized controlled trial

Note. From "Fertility Preservation in Women of Reproductive Age With Cancer," by J.F. McLaren and G.W. Bates, 2012, *American Journal of Obstetrics and Gynecology, 207*, p. 456. doi:10.1016/j.ajog.2012.08.013. Copyright 2012 by Elsevier. Reprinted with permission.

Embryo cryopreservation is the most established of the fertility preservation methods for women. It has some drawbacks that may make it impossible for some women, especially those with hormone-dependent cancers or when treatment cannot be delayed for any length of time. It also requires the participation of a male partner or sperm donor, and this additional barrier may prevent some women, particularly those who are younger, from participating.

The ovaries must be hyperstimulated to create an embryo. This requires large doses of hormones, making it inappropriate for women with hormone-dependent cancers. It also usually means waiting for a certain point in the woman's menstrual cycle to begin the stimulation, further increasing the delay to starting cancer treatment. However, new research has shown that stimulation can begin anywhere in the menstrual cycle and that other medications can promote hyperstimulation, including letrozole and tamoxifen, two agents that are used to prevent recurrence in patients with breast cancer (Sönmezer, Türkçüoğlu, Coşkun, & Oktay, 2011). This may be the preferred method of hyperstimulation because it is safer for women with hormone-dependent cancers. Once the ova have been obtained, they are fertilized with the donor/partner sperm, and the embryos are frozen for later implantation into the woman herself or a surrogate.

Success rates of assisted reproductive technology (ART) are continually improving, with estimates that about 40% of embryos are successfully transferred, although this varies by the woman's age and the fertility center (Duffy & Allen, 2009). Some studies have shown that using frozen ova results in declining live birth rates, especially with increasing age of the woman (Moffat et al., 2012). Women may regard fertility preservation as an "insurance policy" and never go back to use frozen ova or embryos, either because they were able to conceive naturally or because their life circumstances changed and they did not want or need them. In one study, only 9% of breast cancer survivors returned to the fertility clinic to use their frozen ova or embryos (Westphal & Wapnir, 2012).

Oocyte cryopreservation is a newer form of fertility preservation for women that does not require the participation of a male donor. However, it does require hyperstimulation of the ovaries and retrieval of the ova. Improved success rates have led to this method of fertility preservation no longer being regarded as experimental (Loren et al., 2013). Because it does not require the cooperation of a male donor, this method is suitable for younger women and single women. Success rates for this procedure are about a quarter of those for traditional in vitro fertilization (Duffy & Allen, 2009).

Ovarian tissue preservation is an experimental method of surgically removing part of the ovary and freezing it until after treatment when it can be placed back into the woman's body. Much like testicular tissue cryopreservation, there are concerns about reintroducing cancer cells into the woman. Successful pregnancies have been reported, but these are limited, and the ratio of attempts to successes is unknown (Bastings, Beerendonk, Westphal, Braat, & Peek, 2013).

Ovarian suppression using gonadotropin-releasing hormone agonists has not been shown to be effective in preserving fertility. ASCO guidelines state that this is not an effective method but may be used in urgent situations and preferably as part of a clinical trial (Loren et al., 2013).

Experiences of Young Adults With Fertility Preservation

Despite universal agreement that individuals with cancer of reproductive age should receive information about the risks of cancer treatment on future fertility as well as information about fertility preservation, the reality is that many do not (Tschudin & Bitzer, 2009). Cancer in this population has been described as a biologic disruption; being diagnosed as a young adult challenges assumptions about life plans and the future. Fertility issues are seen as biographical accelerators for those with cancer, as young adults in relationships are forced to initiate discussions about issues that would normally be dealt with at a later stage of the relationship. Cancer also can be a biographical stressor in that it forces those in partnered relationships to talk about reproduction when they had not done so before (Barbour, Porter, Peddie, & Bhattacharya, 2013).

A history of cancer does not appear to interfere with young adults wanting children. In a landmark study of cancer survivors' attitudes toward having children (Schover, Rybicki, Martin, & Bringelsen, 1999), researchers found that 76% wanted children of their own. Half of the 283 survivors who participated in the study believed that their fertility had been impaired by the treatment they received, and only 6% had participated in any form of fertility preservation. When asked about the impact of cancer treatment on children they might have in the future, 19% were worried that the health of their children might be impaired by the treatment they received for cancer, and 18% of the women were afraid that becoming pregnant might trigger a recurrence of their cancer. Just more than half of the participants (57%) had received information about fertility at the time of diagnosis, and 24% of the men had banked sperm.

Although that study may be slightly dated, more recent research does not suggest much improvement. In a California study of female cancer survivors (Niemasik et al., 2012), 29% were told not to think about having children because of their poor prognosis. They were told that there was a risk that they could pass their cancer on to their future children. Those who already had a child believed that this played a role in not being informed about fertility preservation. The healthcare providers they talked with appeared uncomfortable and focused on the negatives about fertility preservation, potentially scaring the young women. In this study, just 12.2% recalled receiving information about fertility preservation. Another study suggested that young women are still not getting the information they need. Gorman, Bailey, Pierce, and Su (2012) reported that the young women in their study were hopeful but worried about future fertility. They were frustrated by their lack of choice or control and wanted better information and continuity of care. These women also stated that fertility problems cause relationship challenges.

Another study from the United Kingdom showed a distinction between male and female survivors (Wilkes, Coulson, Crosland, Rubin, & Stewart, 2010). Young men were presented with information about sperm banking routinely and as a matter of course. In comparison, for women, information about impact on fertility was minimized, and the urgency of starting treatment was stressed. Of additional note from this study was the desire for discussion about fertility not just at diagnosis but along the treatment trajectory so that they could talk about it at different stages of their lives.

A more positive perspective was reported in another study from California (Letourneau et al., 2012). In this large retrospective study, more than 1,000 women were asked to recall their experience. Of these women, 61% were counseled by their oncologist and a further 5% were referred to a fertility specialist, which in this study was shown to reduce later regret. However, only 5% pursued fertility preservation.

In a study comparing the experiences of young women in 2004 and 2011, improvements over time were seen, with a much larger percentage of women given information about fertility preservation before treatment started (38% in 2004 vs. 68.9% in 2011). However, dissatisfaction with the information provided was still high (58.9% in 2004 vs. 50% in 2011) (Yeomanson, Morgan, & Pacey, 2013).

The pressure to make a decision about fertility preservation at the time of diagnosis is very difficult (Crawshaw, Glaser, Hale, & Sloper, 2009). Patients have to absorb critical information and are at risk of being overwhelmed by information overload (Peddie et al., 2012). The information provided can be scary for some, and most young adults feel overwhelmed by the information. This may be worse for women than for men. Young men report that the process of sperm banking is clear and straightforward (Crawshaw et al., 2009), whereas young women have multiple factors to consider, including significant financial costs that are often presented in vague terms, thereby further complicating the decision that has to be made (Hill et al., 2012).

Young adults reported feeling pressure at having to make a decision about future parenthood at the same time as they are making life-altering decisions about treatment (Crawshaw et al., 2009). For younger individuals, even thinking about future parenthood is too theoretical to consider properly. For many, the cancer diagnosis and subsequent treatment is a journey of great uncertainty, and the impact on fertility is an additional source of uncertainty (Halliday & Boughton, 2011).

Of importance too is what young adults know about their fertility status after treatment. This has implications for relationships, contraception, and planning for future pregnancy. Young men who have banked sperm have some assurance that they can father children in the future. However, young women who have not pursued fertility preservation have less certainty and may not know where to go to find out about their fertility status (Wright, Coad, Morgan, Stark, & Cable, 2013). Knowing their fertility status is important for many, as it can influence present and future romantic relationships (Gorman et al., 2012).

Knowing about reproductive health outside of fertility is important also. Some young adult survivors may assume that they are infertile and do not bother with contraception. However, they are at risk for sexually transmitted infections and may be fertile despite their assumptions.

Decision Making About Fertility Preservation

The offer of fertility preservation confers hope to young adults newly diagnosed with cancer (Gracia & Jeruss, 2013), especially when it is provided by oncology care providers (Crawshaw et al., 2009). For some women, fertility is related to femininity and female identity (Penrose, Beatty, Mattiske, & Koczwara, 2012), and loss of reproductive potential may be experienced as a loss of self and expected role. When presented with the option of fertility preservation, women must weigh their desire for children against the risks of delaying treatment and potentially affecting the outcome of cancer treatment (Duffy & Allen, 2009). Questions about future fertility also may be seen in the context of the generalized uncertainty that colors the cancer experience. Women may not be entirely certain that they will never bear a biologic child, and if they do become pregnant, they experience uncertainty about the effects of their cancer treatment on the health of the fetus (Halliday & Boughton, 2011).

The need for adjuvant therapy adds to the complexity of fertility-related matters. When women were asked about their feelings toward having chemotherapy and its impact on fertility, the majority stated that cure remained their highest priority. Only 8% responded they would refuse chemotherapy to protect their fertility (Senkus et al., 2014). Younger age, having chemotherapy, and not having children already were associated with concerns about future fertility in another large study (Ruddy et al., 2014). In this study, 1% of those surveyed considered not taking adjuvant endocrine therapy, 3% did not take it when offered, and 11% considered taking endocrine therapy for less than the recommended five years. Just 10% of the women in this study had used fertility preservation.

In a study of young women with cancer who were eligible for fertility preservation (Hershberger, Finnegan, Pierce, & Scoccia, 2013), researchers discovered that these women felt overwhelmed and that the realization that treatment could cause infertility made the diagnosis real. They described being able to see themselves overcoming the cancer, but the loss of fertility was more uncertain and was the cause of grief and heartache. In deciding whether to proceed with fertility preservation, women undertook a number of actions, including gathering as much information as possible and considering prior life experiences and personal values. Women found it stressful to have to make important decisions in a very short time frame while under significant stress. At the same time, they had to weigh the financial costs of the procedures, most of which were not covered by insurance. These issues were echoed in a study from Canada, which additionally identified the challenge for single women to find a sperm donor, a factor that was seen as a barrier to fertility preservation (Yee, Abrol, McDonald, Tonelli, & Liu, 2012). The women in this study also stated that they wanted to preserve their fertility to prevent future regret.

Regret is a theme of some studies about decision making regarding fertility preservation. In a longitudinal study of Australian women with breast cancer, some women who had earlier stated that fertility loss was not an important issue for them changed their minds and later expressed regret that they had not done anything to preserve fertility (Connell, Patterson, & Newman, 2006). Feeling rushed into treatment removed choices for women in another study, and they too expressed regret about lost opportunity (Lee et al., 2011). Long-term survivors may be left with distress related to the interruption of their life plans, particularly those of creating a family with children. Canada and Schover (2012) described increased distress in a study of 240 long-term survivors (more than 10 years). These women experienced intrusive thoughts, used avoidance strategies to reduce distress when reminded of their infertility, and had less relationship and sexual satisfaction. Women who were childless experienced the worst distress, those with adopted children or stepchildren experienced intermediate levels, and women who had children were the least distressed. Decisional regret is associated with not being referred for fertility preservation and also not being able to afford the procedures (Mersereau et al., 2013). For women who are not able to conceive after cancer treatment, their sorrow may be prolonged and they may experience disenfranchised grief that is not validated by family and friends (Kirkman et al., 2014).

For men, fertility may be associated with their self-identity as men. Crawshaw (2013) described the experiences of male cancer survivors with altered fertility in relationship to the perceived stigma of not being able to father children, as well as the reactions of other men joking about sperm banking. The men in this study regarded having banked sperm as part of themselves that could "do the job" if they are not able to.

Being able to make a decision about preserving fertility also may provide a sense of control in a situation where very little control exists (Crawshaw et al., 2009). However, this control may be usurped by others, including parents. Crawshaw et al. (2009) described the instance of a young man who was pressured by his father to bank his sperm, even though he did not want to. The young man described crying for a day and refusing any treatments until his father relented and accepted his decision.

The major factors influencing decision making for young adults are provider related. If oncology care providers do not raise the topic, young adults may not know that their fertility may be affected. If care providers suggest through verbal and nonverbal communication that this is not important or possible, patients are denied the opportunity to ask questions or seek further information. Young adults should have the autonomy to decide whether they want to consider delaying treatment to preserve their fertility. It also is important to recognize that decision making is not a static, solitary event but rather a fluid state as patients progress through various stages along the cancer trajectory. It also is not always a straightforward decision for patients but rather one with many caveats and situational factors that are taken into account (Gardino, Jeruss, & Woodruff, 2010). Young adults have stated that they received very little support as they tried to make a decision (Corney & Swinglehurst, 2014) and that counseling would have been helpful at the time (Hill et al., 2012). Women with breast cancer identified the need for multidisciplinary care, including oncologists, fertility specialists, psychologists, counselors, primary care providers, and specialist nurses, to support them through the spectrum of postdiagnosis challenges (Kirkman et al., 2013).

Attitudes and Practices of Oncology Care Providers

ASCO guidelines clearly state that all oncology care providers have a duty to discuss the impact of cancer treatment on fertility, as well as fertility preservation opportunities (Loren et al., 2013). Despite this, communication regarding the topic is not consistent or even well done. A number of studies have described a lack of information at or after diagnosis and poor communication including the perception on the part of the patient that the oncology care provider was uncomfortable or that he or she seemed to lack knowledge on the topic or dissuaded the patient from considering fertility preservation. Patients place value in the opinion of their oncology care providers, especially soon after diagnosis (Snyder & Tate, 2013). Some oncologists delay talking to patients about fertility until they are older and seen as "ready" to have children of their own, but this is often too late if fertility has been compromised (Gorman et al., 2012). However, when oncology care providers fail to discuss these issues, they are seen by the young adults as unimportant (Duffy & Allen, 2009).

A recent study on the confidence of oncologists in their knowledge about fertility issues in young women with cancer (Duffy, Allen, Dube, & Dickersin, 2012) found that oncologists lack knowledge about fertility issues for women with breast cancer. Only 58% of those surveyed felt a high sense of responsibility to discuss fertility with patients. Just 18% had resources available for patients, and 5% reported using other sources, including social workers, nurse practitioners, or a printed list of websites that had information. Knowledge, and confidence in that knowledge, was low, with just 61.4% reporting that they knew about the risk to future fertility of the medications that they prescribed most often. Less than 25% of respondents had knowledge about fertility preservation methods.

Many young women are unaware of their fertility status at the end of treatment (Wright et al., 2013). This can have significant impact on their future, including unintended pregnancy or relationship problems when they experience difficulty conceiving later.

A study from the United Kingdom reported that although oncologists thought that fertility preservation was an issue primarily for female patients, they felt knowledgeable only about sperm banking. Just 38% of those surveyed routinely provided their patients with printed material on the topic, and one-third did not usually refer their patients to a fertility specialist, even those who had questions about fertility preservation (Adams, Hill, & Watson, 2013). Peddie et al. (2012) highlighted significant problems in how healthcare providers counseled young adults. Participants reported that they were told distressing stories about poor outcomes for those who had pursued fertility preservation before treatment. They stated that the experimental nature of fertility preservation was stressed and that while the men were told about sperm banking, women were told that their treatment needed to start urgently and that they did not have time to pursue fertility preservation. The healthcare professionals who were interviewed for this study had limited knowledge about fertility preservation and also made assumptions about the preferences of their young adult patients.

How information is presented to young adults is important. Gender may play a role, with healthcare providers discussing fertility with men more than with women (Armuand et al., 2012). Barriers to the provision of information about the impact of treatment on fertility or fertility preservation include lack of knowledge on the part of the oncology provider, discomfort with the topic, time constraints, not seeing the issue as important, and a poor prognosis for the patient. Paternalism also is involved, with some physicians stating that treatment decisions are complex and difficult to make and that adding the burden of weighing fertility in the decision process is not appropriate (Duffy & Allen, 2009). For some oncologists, the reluctance to discuss the loss of fertility may stem from their expectation that first-line therapy would not affect fertility but that for those who do not go into remission, second-line therapy is likely to have a negative impact (Peddie et al., 2012).

Recommendations from the Barcelona consensus meeting (Martínez et al., 2013) included the responsibility for oncology care providers to impart realistic information about fertility preservation, including not being overly optimistic about success and providing supportive care for patients' emotional needs. Early referral to a fertility specialist also is recommended, which would, in part, alleviate oncology care providers from the burden of keeping up with the latest evidence about fertility preservation techniques. Findings from studies have suggested that some patients want to have a discussion about fertility more than once (Gorman et al., 2012). Multiple opportunities exist along the care and treatment trajectory where this discussion can be held (Gardino et al., 2010).

Ethical Issues

ART has advanced greatly in the past few years along with improved survival rates for young adults with cancer. Unlike using ART in the noncancer population, where decisions made are acted upon quickly, decisions about using cryopreserved gametes in the case of fertility preservation for young adults with cancer are often made years after retrieval. This presents some unique ethical challenges.

There are more questions than answers for patients considering the ethical challenges inherent in fertility preservation (Shah, Goldman, & Fisseha, 2011). First, is there an increased risk of cancer for the children of cancer survivors? The evidence suggests that no increased risk exists (Shah et al., 2011). There also are issues related to the mortality of the parent with cancer who may leave behind a child or children. However, the risk of premature death exists for everyone; this is not unique to cancer survivors. Attention should be paid by all who cryopreserve reproductive tissues about disposition of this material in the future. It is widely accepted that ova or sperm that are frozen belong to the person from whose body they originated and that person has the sole responsibility to authorize disposal of the tissue. However, this may pose an ethical dilemma when that person dies. Shah et al. (2011) noted that many fertility clinics have contracts with specific content about such decisions that are legally binding. A caution has been raised that consent to fertility preservation should also include understanding of the future use of frozen ova or sperm. Unfortunately, this is not always the case, especially under the time constraints inherent in fertility preservation for young adults with cancer (Quinn & Vadaparampil, 2013).

How to Help the Young Adult With Cancer

Fertility preservation is important to young adults, but their access to services is limited by a number of factors. Some of these are systemic, outside the scope of the individual healthcare provider, and need to be addressed at a policy or state level. For example, some states in the United States have no practicing board-certified fertility specialists (Knapp, Quinn, Rapalo, & Woodworth, 2012).

Despite clear guidelines from ASCO, there are still healthcare providers who do not talk to young adults about the impact of treatment on fertility or who do not offer a referral to a fertility specialist. In some instances, confusion exists about who should or who has talked to the patient. The oncologist may think that the nurse has had the conversation, and the nurse may assume that the oncologist has already done so. The pharmacist may think that it is the oncologist's responsibility. Ultimately, the patient is denied the opportunity to learn about a life-altering side effect of treatment. Evidence from multiple studies has shown that patients often do not recall having a conversation about fertility effects or fertility preservation. This may be because the information is provided at the time of diagnosis when the newly diagnosed patient is in crisis and is not able to retain much information.

One suggested solution is to create policy so that all healthcare providers share in the responsibility of providing fertility-related information. ASCO guidelines (Loren et al., 2013) clearly state that all oncology care providers should be talking to patients about fertility concerns, and these guidelines can form the basis of institutional policy. An innovative program was described by Vadaparampil, Hutchins, and Quinn (2013) in which oncology nurses are trained to provide targeted information to young adult patients. The program, Educating Nurses about Reproductive Issues in Cancer Healthcare (ENRICH), is a distance-learning program consisting of 10 weekly modules. The program addresses not just the learning needs of individual practitioners but also promotes support and change at the institutional level.

Another initiative from this group identified a five-step process to ensure that all eligible patients receive a referral to a fertility specialist (Quinn et al., 2011). Step 1 involved identifying barriers to communicating with patients. Step 2 encompassed educational sessions to address the identified barrier of lack of knowledge. Step 3 was the creation of a referral relationship with an academic fertility specialist practice. This included a dedicated telephone line at the fertility clinic that facilitated a telephone call with a fertility specialist within 24 hours and an appointment for a patient within 48 hours. Step 4 was a pilot study to evaluate a brochure for patients that resulted in a ninefold increase in calls to the fertility clinic over a 12-month period. Finally, step 5 was the inclusion of two questions in the electronic patient health history that all new patients complete. One question asked if the patient had all the children he or she wished to have, and the second asked if the patient would like a referral to a fertility specialist. The response to these questions acted as a prompt to the treating oncologist.

The Fertile Hope Centers of Excellence Program encourages cancer centers to develop strategies to increase the uptake of fertility preservation services (Reinecke et al., 2012). The criteria include professional education, patient education, notification procedures, referrals, and policy development. One of the cancer centers, the Robert H. Lurie Comprehensive Cancer Center of Northwestern University, created fertility screens for its electronic health record. The first screen asks if the patient has been informed about the impact of treatment on his or her fertility. If the answer is yes, a second screen asks if the patient wants information about fertility preservation. If the answer to that question is yes, a referral to a fertility navigator is made automatically. The Oregon Health and Science University has a similar system that also generates printed educational material for patients as well as referral forms.

Cancer Council Australia has a decision aid for young women with cancer (www.cancer.org.au/content/pdf/AboutCancer/OnlineResources/Decision _Aid_breastcancer_fertility_%20June2011.pdf). An evaluation of this document demonstrated that those who read it experienced reduced decisional conflict and regret and showed improved knowledge (Peate et al., 2012).

An additional barrier is the lack of insurance coverage for fertility preservation procedures. The costs for these are prohibitive for most people, especially young adults. While some states mandate coverage for infertility treatments, definitions of infertility do not apply to those with cancer. For example, infertility is defined as not being able to conceive after one year of unprotected intercourse. This obviously does not apply to young adults who want to freeze their eggs before treatment (Knapp et al., 2012).

The following websites may be helpful to both oncology care providers and patients for information and support.
- American Society for Reproductive Medicine: www.asrm.org
- Livestrong Fertility: www.livestrong.org/we-can-help/fertility-services
- MyOncofertility: www.myoncofertility.org
- Oncofertility Consortium: www.oncofertility.northwestern.edu
- Save My Fertility: www.savemyfertility.org

Conclusion

Fertility preservation is a constantly evolving field, and oncology care providers may struggle to keep up with the latest advances. It is also challenging and time consuming to explain the various choices to patients and to know with certainty that the information is accurate and valid. But young adult patients need to know this information, and to not tell them about the impact of treatment on future fertility is neglectful. A referral to a trusted fertility specialist will facilitate accurate information for patients and reduce the amount of regret they may have in the future. Concerns about patients refusing lifesaving treatment to protect fertility are unfounded. Patients will be grateful for the opportunity to explore what can be done, now and in the future, to preserve their fertility.

References

Adams, E., Hill, E., & Watson, E. (2013). Fertility preservation in cancer survivors: A national survey of oncologists' current knowledge, practice and attitudes. *British Journal of Cancer, 108,* 1602–1615. doi:10.1038/bjc.2013.139

Armuand, G.M., Rodriguez-Wallberg, K.A., Wettergren, L., Ahlgren, J., Enblad, G., Höglund, M., & Lampic, C. (2012). Sex differences in fertility-related information received by young adult cancer survivors. *Journal of Clinical Oncology, 30,* 2147–2153. doi:10.1200/JCO.2011.40.6470

Barbour, R.S., Porter, M.A., Peddie, V.L., & Bhattacharya, S. (2013). Counselling in the context of fertility and cancer: Some sociological insights. *Human Fertility, 16,* 54–58. doi:10.3109/14647273.2013.775512

Bastings, L., Beerendonk, C.C.M., Westphal, J.R., Braat, D.D.M., & Peek, R. (2013). Cryopreservation and autotransplantation of ovarian tissue in cancer patients: Is it safe? *Journal of Adolescent and Young Adult Oncology, 2,* 31–34. doi:10.1089/jayao.2012.0017

Berookhim, B.M., & Mulhall, J.P. (2014). Outcomes of operative sperm retrieval strategies for fertility preservation among males scheduled to undergo cancer treatment. *Fertility and Sterility, 101,* 805–811. doi:10.1016/j.fertnstert.2013.11.122

Canada, A.L., & Schover, L.R. (2012). The psychosocial impact of interrupted childbearing in long-term female cancer survivors. *Psycho-Oncology, 21,* 134–143. doi:10.1002/pon.1875

Connell, S., Patterson, C., & Newman, B. (2006). A qualitative analysis of reproductive issues raised by young Australian women with breast cancer. *Health Care for Women International, 27,* 94–110. doi:10.1080/07399330500377580

Corney, R.H., & Swinglehurst, A.J. (2014). Young childless women with breast cancer in the UK: A qualitative study of their fertility-related experiences, options, and the information given by health professionals. *Psycho-Oncology, 23,* 20–26. doi:10.1002/pon.3365

Crawshaw, M. (2013). Male coping with cancer-fertility issues: Putting the "social" into biopsychosocial approaches. *Reproductive BioMedicine Online, 27,* 261–270. doi:10.1016/j.rbmo.2013.04.017

Crawshaw, M.A., Glaser, A.W., Hale, J.P., & Sloper, P. (2009). Male and female experiences of having fertility matters raised alongside a cancer diagnosis during the teenage and young adult years. *European Journal of Cancer Care, 18,* 381–390. doi:10.1111/j.1365-2354.2008.01003.x

Duffy, C., & Allen, S. (2009). Medical and psychosocial aspects of fertility after cancer. *Cancer Journal, 15,* 27–33. doi:10.1097/PPO.0b013e3181976602

Duffy, C., Allen, S.M., Dube, C., & Dickersin, K. (2012). Oncologists' confidence in knowledge of fertility issues for young women with cancer. *Journal of Cancer Education, 27,* 369–376. Retrieved from http://www.ncbi.nlm.nih.gov/pmc/articles/PMC3352969

Gardino, S.L., Jeruss, J.S., & Woodruff, T.K. (2010). Using decision trees to enhance interdisciplinary team work: The case of oncofertility. *Journal of Assisted Reproduction and Genetics, 27,* 227–231. doi:10.1007/s10815-010-9413-8

Gorman, J.R., Bailey, S., Pierce, J.P., & Su, H.I. (2012). How do you feel about fertility and parenthood? The voices of young female cancer survivors. *Journal of Cancer Survivorship, 6,* 200–209. Retrieved from http://www.ncbi.nlm.nih.gov/pmc/articles/PMC3667153

Gospodarowicz, M. (2008). Testicular cancer patients: Considerations in long-term follow-up. *Hematology/Oncology Clinics of North America, 22,* 245–255. doi:10.1016/j.hoc.2008.01.003

Gracia, C.R., & Jeruss, J.S. (2013). Lives in the balance: Women with cancer and the right to fertility care. *Journal of Clinical Oncology, 31,* 668–669. doi:10.1200/JCO.2012.47.5798

Halliday, L.E., & Boughton, M.A. (2011). Exploring the concept of uncertain fertility, reproduction and motherhood after cancer in young adult women. *Nursing Inquiry, 18,* 135–142. doi:10.1111/j.1440-1800.2011.00532.x

Hershberger, P.E., Finnegan, L., Pierce, P.F., & Scoccia, B. (2013). The decision-making process of young adult women with cancer who considered fertility cryopreservation. *Journal of Obstetric, Gynecologic, and Neonatal Nursing, 42,* 59–69. doi:10.1111/j.1552-6909.2012.01426.x

Hill, K.A., Nadler, T., Mandel, R., Burlein-Hall, S., Librach, C., Glass, K., & Warner, E. (2012). Experience of young women diagnosed with breast cancer who undergo fertility preservation consultation. *Clinical Breast Cancer, 12,* 127–132. doi:10.1016/j.clbc.2012.01.002

Johnson, R.H., & Kroon, L. (2013). Optimizing fertility preservation practices for adolescent and young adult cancer patients. *Journal of the National Comprehensive Cancer Network, 11,* 71–77. Retrieved from http://www.jnccn.org/content/11/1/71.long

Katz, D., Kolon, T., Feldman, D., & Mulhall, J. (2013). Fertility preservation strategies for male patients with cancer. *Nature Reviews Urology, 10,* 463–472. doi:10.1038/nrurol.2013.145

Kenney, L.B., Cohen, L.E., Shnorhavorian, M., Metzger, M.L., Lockart, B., Hijiya, N., ... Meacham, L. (2012). Male reproductive health after childhood, adolescent, and young adult cancers: A report from the Children's Oncology Group. *Journal of Clinical Oncology, 30,* 3408–3416. doi:10.1200/JCO.2011.38.6938

Kesic, V. (2008). Fertility after the treatment of gynecologic tumors. In A. Surbone, F. Peccatori, & N. Pavlidis (Eds.), *Recent Results in Cancer Research: Vol. 178. Cancer and pregnancy* (pp. 79–95). doi:10.1007/978-3-540-71274-9_9

Kirkman, M., Stern, C., Neil, S., Winship, I., Mann, G.B., Shanahan, K., ... Fisher, J.R.W. (2013). Fertility management after breast cancer diagnosis: A qualitative investigation of women's experiences of and recommendations for professional care. *Health Care for Women International, 34,* 50–67. doi:10.1080/07399332.2012.735729

Kirkman, M., Winship, I., Stern, C., Neil, S., Mann, G.B., & Fisher, J.R.W. (2014). Women's reflections on fertility and motherhood after breast cancer and its treatment. *European Journal of Cancer Care, 23,* 502–513. doi:10.1111/ecc.12163

Knapp, C.A., Quinn, G.P., Rapalo, D., & Woodworth, L. (2012). Patient provider communication and reproductive health. In G.P. Quinn & S.T. Vadaparampil (Eds.), *Advances in Experimental Medicine and Biology: Vol. 732. Reproductive health and cancer in adolescents and young adults* (pp. 175–185). doi:10.1007/978-94-007-2492-1_14

Lee, R.J., Wakefield, A., Foy, S., Howell, S.J., Wardley, A.M., & Armstrong, A.C. (2011). Facilitating reproductive choices: The impact of health services on the experiences of young women with breast cancer. *Psycho-Oncology, 20,* 1044–1052. doi:10.1002/pon.1826

Letourneau, J.M., Ebbel, E.E., Katz, P.P., Katz, A., Ai, W.Z., Chien, A.J., ... Rosen, M.P. (2012). Pretreatment fertility counseling and fertility preservation improve quality of life in reproductive age women with cancer. *Cancer, 118,* 1710–1717. doi:10.1002/cncr.26459

Loren, A.W., Mangu, P.B., Beck, L.N., Brennan, L., Magdalinski, A.J., Partridge, A.H., ... Oktay, K. (2013). Fertility preservation for patients with cancer: American Society of Clinical Oncology clinical practice guideline update. *Journal of Clinical Oncology, 31,* 2500–2510. doi:10.1200/JCO.2013.49.2678

Martínez, F., Devesa, M., Coroleu, B., Tur, R., González, C., Boada, M., ... Barri, P.N. (2013). Cancer and fertility preservation: Barcelona consensus meeting. *Gynecological Endocrinology, 29,* 285–291. doi:10.3109/09513590.2012.743019

Mersereau, J.E., Goodman, L.R., Deal, A.M., Gorman, J.R., Whitcomb, B.W., & Su, H.I. (2013). To preserve or not to preserve: How difficult is the decision about fertility preservation? *Cancer, 119,* 4044–4050. doi:10.1002/cncr.28317

Moffat, R., de Geyter, C., Myrick, M.E., Schmid, S.M., Sattmann, C., Tschudin, S., ... Güth, U. (2012). Young women with breast cancer: How many are actually candidates for fertility preservation? *Archives of Gynecology and Obstetrics, 286,* 1521–1527. doi:10.1007/s00404-012-2457-5

National Comprehensive Cancer Network. (2014). *NCCN Clinical Practice Guidelines in Oncology (NCCN Guidelines®): Adolescent and young adult (AYA) oncology* [v.2.2015]. Retrieved from http://www.nccn.org/professionals/physician_gls/pdf/aya.pdf

Neal, M.S., Nagel, K., Duckworth, J., Bissessar, H., Fischer, M.A., Portwine, C., ... Barr, R.D. (2007). Effectiveness of sperm banking in adolescents and young adults with cancer. *Cancer, 110,* 1125–1129. doi:10.1002/cncr.22889

Niemasik, E.E., Letourneau, J., Dohan, D., Katz, A., Melisko, M., Rugo, H., & Rosen, M. (2012). Patient perceptions of reproductive health counseling at the time of cancer diagnosis: A qualitative study of female California cancer survivors. *Journal of Cancer Survivorship, 6,* 324–332. doi:10.1007/s11764-012-0227-9

Olatunbosun, O., & Zhu, L. (2012). The role of sperm banking in fertility preservation. *Clinical and Experimental Obstetrics and Gynecology, 39,* 283–287.

Peate, M., Meiser, B., Cheah, B.C., Saunders, C., Butow, P., Thewes, B., ... Friedlander, M. (2012). Making hard choices easier: A prospective, multicentre study to assess the efficacy of a fertility-related decision aid in young women with early-stage breast cancer. *British Journal of Cancer, 106,* 1053–1061. doi:10.1038/bjc.2012.61

Peddie, V.L., Porter, M.A., Barbour, R., Culligan, D., MacDonald, G., King, D., ... Bhattacharya, S. (2012). Factors affecting decision making about fertility preservation after cancer diagnosis: A qualitative study. *BJOG: An International Journal of Obstetrics and Gynaecology, 119,* 1049–1057. doi:10.1111/j.1471-0528.2012.03368.x

Penrose, R., Beatty, L., Mattiske, J., & Koczwara, B. (2012). Fertility and cancer—A qualitative study of Australian cancer survivors. *Supportive Care in Cancer, 20,* 1259–1265. doi:10.1007/s00520-011-1212-y

Quinn, G.P., & Vadaparampil, S.T. (2013). More research, more responsibility: The expansion of duty to warn in cancer patients considering fertility preservation. *American Journal of Obstetrics and Gynecology, 209,* 98–102. doi:10.1016/j.ajog.2013.02.031

Quinn, G.P., Vadaparampil, S.T., Gwede, C.K., Reinecke, J.D., Mason, T.M., & Silva, C. (2011). Developing a referral system for fertility preservation among patients with newly diagnosed cancer. *Journal of the National Comprehensive Cancer Network, 9,* 1219–1225. Retrieved from http://www.jnccn.org/content/9/11/1219.long

Reinecke, J.D., Kelvin, J.F., Arvey, S.R., Quinn, G.P., Levine, J., Beck, L.N., & Miller, A. (2012). Implementing a systematic approach to meeting patients' cancer and fertility needs: A review of the Fertile Hope Centers of Excellence program. *Journal of Oncology Practice, 8,* 303–308. doi:10.1200/JOP.2011.000452

Ruddy, K.J., & Partridge, A.H. (2012). Fertility (male and female) and menopause. *Journal of Clinical Oncology, 30,* 3705–3711. doi:10.1200/JCO.2012.42.1966

Ruddy, K.J., Gelber, S.I., Tamimi, R.M., Ginsburg, E.S., Schapira, L., Come, S.E., ... Partridge, A.H. (2014). Prospective study of fertility concerns and preservation strategies in young women with breast cancer. *Journal of Clinical Oncology, 32,* 1151–1156. doi:10.1200/JCO.2013.52.8877

Salama, M., Winkler, K., Murach, K.R., Seeber, B., Ziehr, S.C., & Wildt, L. (2013). Female fertility loss and preservation: Threats and opportunities. *Annals of Oncology, 24,* 598–608. doi:10.1093/annonc/mds514

Schover, L.R., Rybicki, L.A., Martin, B.A., & Bringelsen, K.A. (1999). Having children after cancer: A pilot survey of survivors' attitudes and experiences. *Cancer, 86,* 697–709. doi:10.1002/(SICI)1097-0142(19990815)86:4<697::AID-CNCR20>3.0.CO;2-J

Senkus, E., Gomez, H., Dirix, L., Jerusalem, G., Murray, E., Van Tienhoven, G., ... Nešković-Konstantinović, Z. (2014). Attitudes of young patients with breast cancer toward fertility loss related to adjuvant systemic therapies. EORTC study 10002 BIG 3-98. *Psycho-Oncology, 23,* 173–182. doi:10.1002/pon.3384

Shah, D.K., Goldman, E., & Fisseha, S. (2011). Medical, ethical, and legal considerations in fertility preservation. *International Journal of Gynaecology and Obstetrics, 115,* 11–15. doi:10.1016/j.ijgo.2011.05.011

Snyder, K.A., & Tate, A.L. (2013). What to do now? How women with breast cancer make fertility preservation decisions. *Journal of Family Planning and Reproductive Health Care, 39,* 172–178. doi:10.1136/jfprhc-2011-100286

Sönmezer, M., Türkçüoğlu, I., Coşkun, U., & Oktay, K. (2011). Random-start controlled ovarian hyperstimulation for emergency fertility preservation in letrozole cycles. *Fertility and Sterility, 95,* 2125.e9–2125.e11. doi:10.1016/j.fertnstert.2011.01.030

Tschudin, S., & Bitzer, J. (2009). Psychological aspects of fertility preservation in men and women affected by cancer and other life-threatening diseases. *Human Reproduction Update, 15,* 587–597. doi:10.1093/humupd/dmp015

Vadaparampil, S.T., Hutchins, N.M., & Quinn, G.P. (2013). Reproductive health in the adolescent and young adult cancer patient: An innovative training program for oncology nurses. *Journal of Cancer Education, 28,* 197–208. Retrieved from http://www.ncbi.nlm.nih.gov/pmc/articles/pmid/23225072

Viatori, M. (2012). Testicular cancer. *Seminars in Oncology Nursing, 28,* 180–189. doi:10.1016/j.soncn.2012.05.007

Wallace, W.H.B. (2011). Oncofertility and preservation of reproductive capacity in children and young adults. *Cancer, 117,* 2301–2310. doi:10.1002/cncr.26045

Westphal, L.M., & Wapnir, I.L. (2012). Integration and safety of fertility preservation in a breast cancer program. *Gynecologic Oncology, 124,* 474–476. doi:10.1016/j.ygyno.2011.11.028

Wilkes, S., Coulson, S., Crosland, A., Rubin, G., & Stewart, J. (2010). Experience of fertility preservation among younger people diagnosed with cancer. *Human Fertility, 13,* 151–158. doi:10.3109/14647273.2010.503359

Wright, C.I., Coad, J., Morgan, S., Stark, D., & Cable, M. (2013). "Just in case": The fertility information needs of teenagers and young adults with cancer. *European Journal of Cancer Care, 23,* 189–198. doi:10.1111/ecc.12137

Yee, S., Abrol, K., McDonald, M., Tonelli, M., & Liu, K.E. (2012). Addressing oncofertility needs: Views of female cancer patients in fertility preservation. *Journal of Psychosocial Oncology, 30,* 331–346. doi:10.1080/07347332.2012.664257

Yeomanson, D.J., Morgan, S., & Pacey, A.A. (2013). Discussing fertility preservation at the time of cancer diagnosis: Dissatisfaction of young females. *Pediatric Blood and Cancer, 60,* 1996–2000. doi:10.1002/pbc.24672

CHAPTER 7
Pregnancy and Parenting

Introduction

For some young adult women, cancer is diagnosed during or after pregnancy. A time of new beginnings is challenged in an unimaginable way for these women and their partner and family. Delayed diagnosis commonly complicates this because it is not a common occurrence and, in the case of breast cancer, may be even more difficult to diagnose because of normal breast changes. However, breast cancer is not the only cancer to be diagnosed in the perinatal period (during and after pregnancy and childbirth); cervical cancer also may be diagnosed during this period. The other common cancers of young adulthood—hematologic and colorectal cancer—may be discovered during this time as well, but breast and cervical cancers are more likely.

This chapter will discuss the incidence and challenges of cancer diagnosed during or after pregnancy and childbirth, as well as the experiences of parenting young children while facing cancer.

Breast Cancer

Cancer occurs in approximately 1 in 1,000 pregnant women, and 7%–15% of breast cancers in premenopausal women are diagnosed during pregnancy (Cardonick, Dougherty, et al., 2010). Pregnancy-associated breast cancer is defined as that occurring during pregnancy and in the first year after the baby is born (Genin et al., 2012). These rates are likely to increase as women delay childbearing until later in life. Breast tissues change during pregnancy in preparation for breast-feeding after birth, and breast-feeding further alters the physiology of these tissues. A woman who feels a lump in her breast may be told by her healthcare provider that what she feels is normal and part of the changes associated with pregnancy or breast-feeding. Many obstetricians have little experience with cancer diagnosed during pregnancy and may not know what to do with a patient who is anxious and confused (Theriault & Litton, 2013). Oncologists, particularly those who specialize in breast cancer, are more familiar with the diagnostic process and treatment options for women found to have breast cancer during or shortly after pregnancy and childbirth.

Any suspicious lump in the breast during pregnancy should be investigated. Mammograms during pregnancy are able to identify suspicious lesions in 90% of pregnant women with invasive breast cancer, and ultrasound also can be helpful in this situation. Shielding of the fetus is recommended if a mammogram is performed in pregnancy (Yang, Dryden, Gwyn, Whitman, & Theriault, 2006). A core biopsy should be performed (rather than fine needle biopsy) to provide enough tissue for hormonal and HER2 analysis (Nye, Huyck, & Gradishar, 2012). The use of sentinel node biopsy is controversial, but it is considered safe as long as blue dye is not used, as this contrast medium has not been tested in this population (Cardonick, Usmani, & Ghaffar, 2010; García-Manero et al., 2009).

The diagnosis of pregnancy-associated breast cancer may precipitate extreme distress for the patient and her family and may be very challenging for the healthcare provider. In these cases there are two patients—the woman and the fetus—and care should be taken to consider the needs of both in treatment decision making. The cancer will be seen as a threat to the woman's life and also as a threat to the fetus. The pregnancy also may be perceived as a threat to the woman's life, and treatment may be seen as a threat to the fetus's well-being and survival (Theriault & Litton, 2013). It is now widely accepted that treatment for pregnancy-associated breast cancer should conform to the standard of treatment for women who are not pregnant, with some cautions. The aim is to control the cancer and prevent systemic spread (García-Manero et al., 2009).

Pregnancy-associated breast cancer has traditionally been characterized by more advanced stage at diagnosis, estrogen receptor negative (Theriault & Litton, 2013), and more likely to overexpress HER2 (Genin et al., 2012). However, overall survival does not differ in these women when compared to nonpregnant women, according to the results of an international study of almost 500 women compared to 865 matched controls (Amant et al., 2013). It is recommended that chemotherapy not be given until the second or third trimester, after development of fetal organs (Lataifeh et al., 2011; Ring et al., 2005). However, surgery (mastectomy or lumpectomy) can be performed safely at any stage of pregnancy, with adjuvant chemotherapy delayed until after the period of organogenesis. Women diagnosed in the first trimester can thus have surgery and delay chemotherapy until later in the pregnancy. Women treated with lumpectomy should delay radiation therapy until after the baby is delivered, as radiation at any stage of pregnancy should be avoided because of toxicity to the fetus (Cardonick, Usmani, et al., 2010; Nye et al., 2012).

Studies have shown that neonatal outcomes after maternal chemotherapy in pregnancy are not adversely affected, and risk of preterm delivery, congenital abnormalities, and low birth weight are no different from outcomes in pregnant women without cancer (Cardonick, Usmani, et al., 2010).

Pregnancy after breast cancer also appears to be safe and may in fact have a protective effect on survival. A study by Córdoba et al. (2012) showed that five-year survival in women pregnant after cancer was 100% compared to 80% in nonpregnant controls. This finding is supported in other studies, including one from Denmark that found that women with breast cancer who had a full-term pregnancy were less likely to die (relative risk 0.73; 95% confidence interval [0.54, 0.99]) than other women with breast cancer (Kroman, Jensen, Wohlfahrt, & Ejlertsen, 2008). This may reflect the "healthy mother effect" in which only women with better prognoses become pregnant and so skew the outcomes. New chemotherapy protocols of reduced duration have been shown to increase life expectancy and enable younger women to consider pregnancy after treatment for breast cancer is over. This study found some small (not statistically significant) increase in adverse events for women who became pregnant within 12 months of diagnosis (Kranick et al., 2010); however, the recommendation is for women to wait two to three years after diagnosis before attempting to get pregnant. With greater awareness and availability of fertility preservation for women with cancer (Ruddy et al., 2014), pregnancy after breast cancer may be more desirable and possible, and evidence of safety should be of comfort and encouragement to young women. Women need to know this so that they can make informed decisions about family planning.

For women with estrogen receptor–positive disease, endocrine manipulation will be needed for upwards of five years after other treatment. This may delay pregnancy and narrow the window of opportunity for pregnancy because of the risk of premature menopause (Christinat & Pagani, 2012; Koczwara, 2008).

Other Cancers

Limited information is available about the risks for and management of pregnancy with other types of cancer. Outcomes for women and neonates after cervical cancer suggest a higher risk for operative delivery, longer hospital stays (more than five days), low and very low birth weight, prematurity, and fetal death (Dalrymple et al., 2005). Recommendations from an international consensus meeting on gynecologic cancer included taking a multidisciplinary approach to management, counseling both parents about the risks of treatment to the fetus and to the pregnant woman, and treating the cancer during pregnancy, including delaying chemotherapy until the second or third trimester (Amant et al., 2009). Delivery should be delayed until after 35 weeks to prevent complications of prematurity.

For women with thyroid cancer diagnosed during pregnancy, radioiodine did not have adverse effects on either the woman or the neonate or subsequent pregnancies and was deemed safe. However, delaying a subsequent pregnancy for a year after radioiodine treatment is recommended (Chow, Yau, Lee, Leung, & Law, 2004).

The Experience of Young Women

Women with breast cancer do get pregnant, purposively and by accident, and their experience of both the pregnancy and cancer is affected. Two lives are affected—and difficult choices must be made. The woman has new life growing inside her, but her own life is being threatened. She may find herself at odds with her healthcare providers; immediate and aggressive treatment will place the well-being of the fetus at risk, but protecting the fetus by delaying treatment may put her life at risk. She also may find herself at odds with her partner and family, who may want her to instead risk the well-being of the fetus, which may be more abstract to them than to her, and do everything she can to potentiate her survival.

Having children of one's own is emotional and symbolic. The desire to have a child does not go away when life is threatened and, in fact, may increase in the face of mortality. Motherhood is a desired and normal state for many women, and having children after a cancer diagnosis may be even more important and meaningful than it was before the illness. This may hold true for men too, despite the fear that many men have when their partner is diagnosed with cancer during pregnancy. These issues were addressed in a study from Israel (Braun, Hasson-Ohayon, Perry, Kaufman, & Uziely, 2005) that found that while couples still wanted to have children after breast cancer, their desire for a large family with many children was modified, and they were not willing to take on too many risks and were happy to settle for a smaller family. The women in this study wanted their existing children to have siblings and to give them a normal life. For the men in the study, the desire for immortality through having children was a motivator for future pregnancies after their partner's cancer.

In a study from Australia (Connell, Patterson, & Newman, 2006), pregnancy was greeted with happiness by some women and with fear by others. Some of the women were concerned about breast-feeding, especially from the affected breast (if lumpectomy had been performed). The women also were concerned about breast changes during lactation and the difficulty of finding a lump in their breast at this time; they were not able to do their usual breast self-examination, and this caused them anxiety. Breast-feeding is possible, even from an irradiated breast, although milk supply will be significantly decreased from that breast. However, it is recommended that women breast-feed if they can, and they should be advised that feeding from one breast is adequate and that the quality of their breast milk is perfect for their baby (Christinat & Pagani, 2012).

Two recent studies have investigated the experience of young women who were diagnosed during pregnancy. The first (Henry, Huang, Sproule, & Cardonick, 2012) found that women diagnosed with different kinds of cancer (i.e., breast, lymphoma, ovarian, melanoma, and other nonspecified) were at highest risk of distress if they had not received fertility assistance to conceive this pregnancy, had been advised to terminate the pregnancy, had a cesarean delivery, were not able to breast-feed, had experienced a recurrence, had further surgery after the pregnancy, or gave birth prematurely. In this study, 51.5% of the women experienced clinical distress. The authors suggested that the additional support and counseling received from a fertility specialist may account for the increased distress among those who did not receive this service. It is interesting that some of the women had been encouraged to terminate the pregnancy; this is not a medical recommendation, and the report does not state if the pressure to terminate came from the healthcare team or family/friends. If it is the former, then deciding to continue the pregnancy against medical advice is likely an important source of stress and distress. Cesarean delivery places additional stress on a woman because it is invasive surgery with an extended recovery period. Distress related to recurrence and further surgery, especially if it is related to the cancer, is another obvious cause of distress. Finally, not being able to breast-feed may be a source of distress to women without a cancer history, and many women feel guilty about this.

The second study (Ives, Musiello, & Saunders, 2012) described the experiences of women diagnosed with breast cancer in the peripartum period (during and after pregnancy). The focus of this report was on the causes of anxiety and stress, both of which were experienced by all the women in the study. High levels of anxiety and stress had an impact on their lives throughout the pregnancy and after the birth of their baby. The anxiety began with the diagnosis of cancer while pregnant, which put them in a position of having to deal with the complexities of their health versus that of the fetus. Concerns about their own health and what treatment might do to the health of the fetus was complicated by what they perceived as conflict between their oncology care providers and their obstetrician related to delivery date and the need to have anticancer treatment. The women felt conflicted as the obstetrician advocated for extending the pregnancy for the sake of fetal maturity and well-being while the oncologist wanted the baby delivered so that the women could have treatment that was precluded by the continued pregnancy. Women who received treatment while pregnant were worried about the effect on the fetus. Some women did not understand what tests they were having and why, and this worried them. They were anxious, as many women are, about the delivery of the baby, and when the obstetrician insisted on a cesarean delivery, this caused further stress if the woman had planned for a natural delivery. If the baby was delivered early and needed to be admitted to the neonatal intensive care unit, anxiety was further compounded. Breast-feeding became a source of stress too—many of the women had to transition the baby to bottle feeding because they needed to start chemotherapy.

A pivotal issue in this study was whether the woman already had children or if this was her first pregnancy. For women who already had children, their priority was to protect themselves and do whatever they could to increase their chances of survival so that they could parent their existing children. Some of these women considered terminating the pregnancy to maximize their chances of survival, although they were torn between this and protecting the future of the fetus. Women who were pregnant for the first time wanted to protect the fetus, but they realized that their health could be adversely affected if they delayed treatment, and this was the inherent source of conflict resulting in distress and high anxiety. In short, women want to protect their children above all else, including their own needs. They experienced stress and anxiety throughout the pregnancy and beyond. They found themselves in situations where there was no right or wrong way, just heartache and the imperative to balance life choices, often when they themselves were young and ill prepared for these sorts of choices.

While women with breast or cervical cancer may have some flexibility in delaying the start of chemotherapy until it is safe for the fetus, women with acute leukemia often do not, and they have to terminate the pregnancy in order to start treatment and save their lives (Schover, 2000). However, some women may choose to terminate the pregnancy even if there is no treatment-related reason to do so. This choice may be made in the context of caring for existing children or out of fear of exposing the fetus to the toxicity of chemotherapy. Little evidence is available to help healthcare providers or patients to deal with this difficult situation.

No recent guidelines exist for the care of pregnant women diagnosed with cancer. An older guideline from the Society of Obstetricians and Gynecologists of Canada (Helewa et al., 2002) confirmed the findings from the more recent literature reported in this chapter. The American Society of Clinical Oncology does not have guidelines on the topic.

Parenting After Cancer

The rigors of treatment for cancer and the late-term effects of treatment on parents have received limited attention in the literature. Much of the focus has been on women with breast cancer.

A study of young women with breast cancer focusing on the role of motherhood is illuminating on many levels (Fisher & O'Connor, 2012). In this study of women with children, breast cancer was experienced as a biographical disruption that had far-reaching consequences. Beginning with diagnosis, the women in this study experienced a range of emotions including disbelief, fear, anger, confusion, denial, depression, and numbness. These young women had to find a way to tell their children about the cancer, which was particularly challenging because despite seeking out information about how to do this, they found little to guide them. Another challenge was that they did not know what to expect in response to their disclosure. They felt out of control and guilty because they could no longer fulfill their roles as mothers because of the demands and aftereffects of treatment. This inability to mother the way they had before the diagnosis was a source of anxiety. They tried as best they could to maintain a sense of normality for their children, and this helped them to link their past and present lives through the actions and routines of everyday care for their children. When they could not care for their children, they found ways for others to do this. Living with breast cancer as a mother with children required reconstruction of their identity, which included thinking about and planning for their children if they do not survive the cancer. This caused them to think about mothering as a time-limited role. Surviving breast cancer was ultimately an empowering experience for these young women, and they emerged with strong feelings about their ability to handle adversity, enhanced self-esteem, and mental strength. This personal growth also involved a reevaluation of needs and priorities and an ability to live in the present and let go of materialistic, financial, and career aspirations.

On a cautionary level, the women in this study reported mostly negative experiences with the healthcare system and healthcare providers (Fisher & O'Connor, 2012). Lack of flexibility in appointment times and the assumption that they could and would neglect their mothering roles to comply with treatment requirements were a source of frustration. They felt that medical professionals objectified them and saw them as patients rather than as women and mothers. This objectification carried through to friends and acquaintances, who the women felt judged them on their altered physical appearance. In response, they alienated themselves. They felt as though others expected them to be or act a certain way and that what they were actually feeling was not validated. Some were not sure what to feel, and they struggled to balance the roles of mother and patient.

A study from Korea (Kim, Ko, & Jun, 2012) reported that being able to focus on the self and the conflict this entailed required delicate balance. The women experienced difficulty taking care of children, which was related to their health, the support they had from family, and the cultural notions of parenting as well as the stigma of cancer in Korean society. The women in this study were also challenged with disclosing their cancer to their children and promoting independence in a timely manner. Finally, they had to envision a different future for themselves and their children in the aftermath of cancer.

Fatherhood after cancer was examined in a literature review (O'Neill, McCaughan, Semple, & Ryan, 2013). The review included six studies, only one of which looked at only men. The findings of this review suggested that fathers' roles have changed over time and now include more complexity, including an active role in the emotional and practical lives of their children rather than a predominantly financial provider role, and in some families the father is the primary care provider. Being a father is now seen as part of masculine identity, and the loss of this role due to the rigors and side effects of treatment may affect identity in much the same ways it does for mothers. It also may affect the children socially and academically. The stereotypical reluctance of men to express and share feelings and seek help is still apparent in the literature; however, this does appear to be changing as men's roles evolve. Much like women, men respond to the diagnosis of cancer with feelings of helplessness. However, having cancer results in a new perspective on their role in the family. For some, the dual roles of husband and father are experienced as stressors as well as resources.

The Effects of Parental Cancer on Children

Studies have looked at the effects of a parent's cancer on children. However, most of them have a mixed sample of school-age and adolescent or older children, which makes it difficult to address the issues for children of young adults (younger than age 35), who are typically school-age or younger.

In a review and meta-synthesis of studies of children (mixed ages) with a parent with nonterminal cancer (Huang, O'Connor, & Lee, 2014), the authors identified five themes from the literature to date: (a) being informed about the cancer, (b) emotional concerns, (c) changes in daily life, (d) seeking factual information, and (e) seeking emotional support. In terms of being informed about the parent's diagnosis of cancer, younger children were given more limited information. However, even when they were not told explicitly, many perceived the bad news before they were told or found out accidentally when they visited the parent in the hospital and saw a sign that said "cancer" or were told by others (such as friends or family members) who did not know that the child had not been told yet. Children reacted to the diagnosis as expected, with shock, worry, fear, anxiety and depression, sadness, and uncertainty. Some cried frequently and some felt guilty, believing that they had done something to cause the cancer. No matter their age, the cancer diagnosis was associated with death, and this caused worry and insecurity about their own future without the parent. Alterations in the parent's physical appearance due to treatment, especially hair loss from chemotherapy, was most disturbing to younger children but affected all children. Separation from the parent during hospitalizations was an additional stressor for some. Their worry extended to thoughts of others in the family getting cancer, including themselves.

When a parent has cancer, changes in the daily life of the family are inevitable. Children may have to give up hobbies, sports, or extracurricular activities for a while. Some children may have to get used to others doing what their parent used to do, and this can be stressful. Children notice the altered behavior of the parent due to treatment, including lack of energy and emotional vulnerability, and some children may try to protect their parents by not sharing their own emotions and altering their own behavior in an attempt to be helpful or minimize conflict with siblings. Over time, many families are able to integrate the changes brought about by cancer and return to some sort of normal life. Some children try to distract themselves from what is happening and keep to themselves and not demand attention.

Seeking information about the cancer applies to older children and adolescents. The literature suggests that younger children have limited needs for information (Huang et al., 2014); these may be met by trusted family members other than parents and teachers at school. Younger children may not have the cognitive ability to actively seek emotional support. The literature reviewed suggests that they may tell their friends that their parent has cancer; however, some are embarrassed and do not want anyone to know, particularly anyone at school, as that may be their only refuge and unaffected place for them (Huang et al., 2014).

Very little research exists on the response to and effects from having a parent with advanced or metastatic cancer. One study (Kennedy & Lloyd-Williams, 2009) of children between the ages of 8 and 18 suggested that this scenario is particularly distressing, as it forces children to face the reality of death. This makes children think about what might happen to them and any siblings after the parent dies. In this study, some parents had not told their children about the severity of their illness. However, they observed behavioral problems in their children that they often ascribed to something else (adolescent rebellion, for example) rather than a response to what the children were seeing and not being told about the cancer. Much like the children of parents with nonterminal cancer, these children used distraction to cope with alterations in routine. Some children reported being closer to their parents, being prepared for independence, and learning to appreciate life (Kennedy & Lloyd-Williams, 2009); it is reasonable to assume that this is more likely to be a response of older children who have the capacity to express this.

Oncology care providers have a duty to assist patients in all aspects of supporting children, but this may be neglected. A study from Australia (Turner et al., 2007) found that women with advanced cancer received very little help from their care providers, and when they did, counselors seemed to have little information for those with advanced cancer who did not have a good chance of long-term survival. One woman in the study found that the counselor was too confrontational when dealing with the topic of the patient's mortality, and this was traumatic for her.

How to Help the Young Adult With Cancer

Talking about the risks inherent in pregnancy with a pregnant woman with cancer requires a great deal of expertise and sensitivity. She will likely be both anxious about her own health and happy about her pregnancy. She may want to know the risks for her own life if she continues the pregnancy, as well as the risks to the fetus if she undergoes treatment. Zanetti-Dällen-bach et al. (2006) suggested that conversations about this occur with privacy and adequate time. Assessing the understanding of the woman and her part-ner (if present) is important to the healthcare provider so that information is presented in a way that the woman can hear and understand what is being told to her. Information should be honest and simple, with ample oppor-tunity provided for questions and clarification. Zanetti-Dällenbach et al. (2006) also recommended that great care be taken in communicating risk to the woman to minimize misunderstandings. They suggested talking about positive outcomes (90 out of 100 women will be cured) as well as negative outcomes (10 out of 100 women will die). They suggested providing abso-lute risk rather than relative risk, as the latter can be misleading, and they also suggested using diagrams and images as much as possible to explain in a visual manner what the woman's risks are.

Zanetti-Dällenbach et al. (2006) further recommended that the woman should be encouraged to express her feelings, and for this reason, they advised that a multidisciplinary team be involved in the patient's care. It is important to offer the woman help in telling others about her cancer, preg-nancy, and treatment plan, as well as to provide her with a referral for sup-portive services as appropriate.

The literature recommends talking openly and honestly with children of all ages about the parent's cancer. Some children prefer to try to live their lives as normally as possible and do not want to engage in activities related to the cancer (e.g., going to the hospital) or to talk about it and share their emotions. This may reflect a desire to protect their parents and lessen their burden (Huang et al., 2014). Women in one study (Turner et al., 2007) wanted a resource that included topics such as reassurance that being hon-est with children was the best thing for them. They wanted practical tips on how to spend more time with their families and how to protect their chil-dren from hurtful comments from others. They also wanted to be reminded that providing children with information was not a onetime event but some-thing that needed to be revisited again and again over time.

Formal programs involving parents and children have been evaluated. An intensive five-session Enhancing Connections Program delivered every other week showed significant improvement in depression, anxiety, and confidence in assisting children among mothers with breast cancer who participated. Mothers and fathers who participated noticed fewer behavioral problems with their children after the program, as well as improvement in the children's mood. The children themselves reported a decrease in cancer-related worry (Lewis, Casey, Brandt, Shands, & Zahlis, 2006). The content of the program included education to help the women with breast cancer to be more aware of the triggers for their own emotions in order to help their child or children, building listening skills, and increasing capacity to assess their child's or children's coping skills.

Another study compared a culturally specific family intervention for African Americans affected by parental cancer with a standard psychoeducational intervention (Davey, Kissil, Harmon, & Hodgson, 2013). Specific attention was paid to unique aspects of African American culture, including focusing on religious faith and kin support, highlighting positives, and encouraging flexibility in family roles. Those in the intervention group showed significantly better communication skills and were more satisfied than the control group. The interactive nature of the intervention coupled with the opportunities to share with others helped to create a sense of community, which is seen as a core facet of African American culture.

Conclusion

Despite the risk to fertility from cancer treatment as discussed in Chapter 6, some women will become pregnant and will need support and guidance as they approach what should be a joyous event with trepidation and fear. Cancer in a young family carries with it significant risk for distress in both parents and children, and the need for support for all members of the family is obvious. Although not many evidence-based interventions are available for these families, at a minimum they should be referred for psychosocial support at any point in the disease trajectory when the need is identified. A routine referral for assessment early in the disease trajectory may be of benefit because some patients may not identify their own risk for problems with coping or may be too busy to report problems.

References

Amant, F., Van Calsteren, K., Halaska, M.J., Beijnen, J., Lagae, L., Hanssens, M., ... du Bois, A. (2009). Gynecologic cancers in pregnancy: Guidelines of an international consensus meeting. *International Journal of Gynecological Cancer, 19*(Suppl. 1), S1–S12. doi:10.1111/IGC.0b013e3181a1d0ec

Amant, F., von Minckwitz, G., Han, S.N., Bontenbal, M., Ring, A., Giermek, J., ... Loibl, S. (2013). Prognosis of women with primary breast cancer diagnosed during pregnancy: Results from an international collaborative study. *Journal of Clinical Oncology, 31*, 2532–2539. doi:10.1200/JCO.2012.45.6335

Braun, M., Hasson-Ohayon, I., Perry, S., Kaufman, B., & Uziely, B. (2005). Motivation for giving birth after breast cancer. *Psycho-Oncology, 14*, 282–296. doi:10.1002/pon.844

Cardonick, E., Dougherty, R., Grana, G., Gilmandyar, D., Ghaffar, S., & Usmani, A. (2010). Breast cancer during pregnancy: Maternal and fetal outcomes. *Cancer Journal, 16*, 76–82. doi:10.1097/PPO.0b013e3181ce46f9

Cardonick, E., Usmani, A., & Ghaffar, S. (2010). Perinatal outcomes of a pregnancy complicated by cancer, including neonatal follow-up after in utero exposure to chemotherapy: Results of an international registry. *American Journal of Clinical Oncology, 33*, 221–228. doi:10.1097/COC.0b013e3181a44ca9

Chow, S.-M., Yau, S., Lee, S.-H., Leung, W.-M., & Law, S.C.K. (2004). Pregnancy outcome after diagnosis of differentiated thyroid carcinoma: No deleterious effect after radioactive iodine treatment. *International Journal of Radiation Oncology, Biology, Physics, 59*, 992–1000. doi:10.1016/j.ijrobp.2003.12.023

Christinat, A., & Pagani, O. (2012). Fertility after breast cancer. *Maturitas, 73*, 191–196. doi:10.1016/j.maturitas.2012.07.013

Connell, S., Patterson, C., & Newman, B. (2006). A qualitative analysis of reproductive issues raised by young Australian women with breast cancer. *Health Care for Women International, 27*, 94–110. doi:10.1080/07399330500377580

Córdoba, O., Bellet, M., Vidal, X., Cortés, J., Llurba, E., Rubio, I.T., & Xercavins, J. (2012). Pregnancy after treatment of breast cancer in young women does not adversely affect the prognosis. *Breast, 21*, 272–275. doi:10.1016/j.breast.2011.10.001

Dalrymple, J.L., Gilbert, W.M., Leiserowitz, G.S., Cress, R., Xing, G., Danielsen, B., & Smith, L.H. (2005). Pregnancy-associated cervical cancer: Obstetric outcomes. *Journal of Maternal-Fetal and Neonatal Medicine, 17*, 269–276. doi:10.1080/14767050500123962

Davey, M., Kissil, K., Harmon, L., & Hodgson, N. (2013). A culturally adapted family intervention for African American families coping with parental cancer: Outcomes of a pilot study. *Psycho-Oncology, 22*, 1572–1580. doi:10.1002/pon.3172

Fisher, C., & O'Connor, M. (2012). "Motherhood" in the context of living with breast cancer. *Cancer Nursing, 35*, 157–163. doi:10.1097/NCC.0b013e31821cadde

García-Manero, M., Royo, M.P., Espinos, J., Pina, L., Alcazar, J.L., & López, G. (2009). Pregnancy associated breast cancer. *European Journal of Surgical Oncology, 35*, 215–218. doi:10.1016/j.ejso.2008.04.010

Genin, A.-S., Lesieur, B., Gligorov, J., Antoine, M., Selleret, L., & Rouzier, R. (2012). Pregnancy-associated breast cancers: Do they differ from other breast cancers in young women? *Breast, 21*, 550–555. doi:10.1016/j.breast.2012.05.002

Helewa, M., Lévesque, P., Provencher, D., Lea, R.H., Rosolowich, V., & Shapiro, H.M. (2002). Breast cancer, pregnancy, and breastfeeding. *Journal of Obstetrics and Gynaecology Canada, 24*, 164–80.

Henry, M., Huang, L.N., Sproule, B.J., & Cardonick, E.H. (2012). The psychological impact of a cancer diagnosed during pregnancy: Determinants of long-term distress. *Psycho-Oncology, 21*, 444–450. doi:10.1002/pon.1926

Huang, X., O'Connor, M., & Lee, S. (2014). School-aged and adolescent children's experience when a parent has non-terminal cancer: A systematic review and meta-synthesis of qualitative studies. *Psycho-Oncology, 23*, 493–506. doi:10.1002/pon.3457

Ives, A., Musiello, T., & Saunders, C. (2012). The experience of pregnancy and early motherhood in women diagnosed with gestational breast cancer. *Psycho-Oncology, 21*, 754–761. doi:10.1002/pon.1970

Kennedy, V.L., & Lloyd-Williams, M. (2009). How children cope when a parent has advanced cancer. *Psycho-Oncology, 18,* 886–892. doi:10.1002/pon.1455

Kim, S., Ko, Y.H., & Jun, E.Y. (2012). The impact of breast cancer on mother–child relationships in Korea. *Psycho-Oncology, 21,* 640–646. doi:10.1002/pon.1941

Koczwara, B. (2008). Addressing fertility needs of breast cancer patients: Oncology perspective. *Expert Review of Anticancer Therapy, 8,* 1323–1330. doi:10.1586/14737140.8.8.1323

Kranick, J.A., Schaefer, C., Rowell, S., Desai, M., Petrek, J.A., Hiatt, R.A., & Senie, R.T. (2010). Is pregnancy after breast cancer safe? *Breast Journal, 16,* 404–411. doi:10.1111/j.1524 -4741.2010.00939.x

Kroman, N., Jensen, M.-B., Wohlfahrt, J., & Ejlertsen, B. (2008). Pregnancy after treatment of breast cancer—A population-based study on behalf of Danish Breast Cancer Cooperative Group. *Acta Oncologica, 47,* 545–549. doi:10.1080/02841860801935491

Lataifeh, I.M., Al Masri, M., Barahmeh, S., Otay, L., Obeidat, N., Badran, O., ... Jaradat, I. (2011). Management of cancer during pregnancy: Obstetric and neonatal outcomes. *International Journal of Gynecological Cancer, 21,* 1159–1164. doi:10.1097/IGC.0b013e31821e73b2

Lewis, F.M., Casey, S.M., Brandt, P.A., Shands, M.E., & Zahlis, E.H. (2006). The enhancing connections program: Pilot study of a cognitive-behavioral intervention for mothers and children affected by breast cancer. *Psycho-Oncology, 15,* 486–497. doi:10.1002/pon.979

Nye, L., Huyck, T.K., & Gradishar, W.J. (2012). Diagnostic and treatment considerations when newly diagnosed breast cancer coincides with pregnancy: A case report and review of literature. *Journal of the National Comprehensive Cancer Network, 10,* 145–148. Retrieved from http://www.jnccn.org/content/10/2/145.long

O'Neill, C., McCaughan, E., Semple, C., & Ryan, A. (2013). Fatherhood and cancer: A commentary on the literature. *European Journal of Cancer Care, 22,* 161–168. doi:10.1111/ecc.12021

Ring, A.E., Smith, I.E., Jones, A., Shannon, C., Galani, E., & Ellis, P.A. (2005). Chemotherapy for breast cancer during pregnancy: An 18-year experience from five London teaching hospitals. *Journal of Clinical Oncology, 23,* 4192–4197. doi:10.1200/JCO.2005.03.038

Ruddy, K.J., Gelber, S.I., Tamimi, R.M., Ginsburg, E.S., Schapira, L., Come, S.E., ... Partridge, A.H. (2014). Prospective study of fertility concerns and preservation strategies in young women with breast cancer. *Journal of Clinical Oncology, 32,* 1151–1156. doi:10.1200/JCO.2013.52.8877

Schover, L.R. (2000). Psychosocial issues associated with cancer in pregnancy. *Seminars in Oncology, 27,* 699–703.

Theriault, R., & Litton, J. (2013). Pregnancy during or after breast cancer diagnosis: What do we know and what do we need to know? *Journal of Clinical Oncology, 31,* 2521–2522. doi:10.1200/JCO.2013.49.7347

Turner, J., Clavarino, A., Yates, P., Hargraves, M., Connors, V., & Hausmann, S. (2007). Development of a resource for parents with advanced cancer: What do parents want? *Palliative and Supportive Care, 5,* 135–145. doi:10.1017/S1478951507070204

Yang, W.T., Dryden, M.J., Gwyn, K., Whitman, G.J., & Theriault, R. (2006). Imaging of breast cancer diagnosed and treated with chemotherapy during pregnancy. *Radiology, 239,* 52–60. doi:10.1148/radiol.2391050083

Zanetti-Dällenbach, R., Tschudin, S., Lapaire, O., Holzgreve, W., Wight, E., & Bitzer, J. (2006). Psychological management of pregnancy-related breast cancer. *Breast, 15*(Suppl. 2), S53–S59. doi:10.1016/S0960-9776(07)70019-X

CHAPTER 8
Family and Friends

Introduction

The diagnosis of a life-threatening disease in a young adult child defies the natural order of life wherein parents are supposed to die before their children. Cancer in the young adult child occurs at a time of transition for both the parents and the young adult; the young adult is transitioning to an independent life and the parents are moving on in their lives with less responsibility for their child. Both the parents and the young adult are experiencing increasing freedom, and this is jeopardized by the illness.

This chapter will describe the challenges to parents and other family members as well as friends of the young adult with cancer as they face the uncertainty inherent in a life-threatening illness. The changes that occur in the parent-child relationship resulting from the illness also will be discussed.

Young Adulthood as a Transitional State

As discussed in Chapter 1, young adulthood is a time of transition. Young adults become more independent with school and career responsibilities, the establishment of primary relationships outside of the family, and a life that becomes in many ways distant from the family of origin. The diagnosis of cancer shatters the fragility of this new life and requires a renegotiation of roles within the family. It may be very difficult for young adults to give up their independence and rely on their parents again for practical, emotional, and financial support as is often necessitated by serious illness. However, it also is difficult for the parents to witness this loss of independence and to experience their young adult child become increasingly dependent on them again.

The Impact of the Cancer Diagnosis

A diagnosis of cancer always results in shock. Additionally, young adults often experience a prolonged delay in diagnosis, as they were told over and over that they were "too young" to have cancer. So when they are finally diagnosed, the reality may seem surreal or even impossible to comprehend. Young adults may not have the capacity to understand the seriousness of the diagnosis; they may have had little to no experience of life-threatening illness in family members or friends and therefore do not fully comprehend what is told to them. Young adults may not have the necessary skills and maturity to deal with the diagnosis and the decisions that have to be made on an ongoing basis about treatment choices, management of the illness, hospital admissions, end-of-life care, and so on. They may also choose to deliberately minimize the seriousness of the diagnosis in an attempt to cope. When parents see this as denial or being out of touch with reality, conflict may ensue.

Some parents may try to shield their child from the severity of the illness and ask healthcare providers to keep this information from the child, despite the fact that the patient is old enough to legally make his or her own treatment decisions. This places healthcare providers in a precarious position and should be avoided. Barling, Stevens, and Davis (2013) described the challenges of young adults in interpreting technical language and needing help from parents who themselves often need assistance in understanding what the information means. This study also described inconsistencies in inclusion of family members in communication about the disease; at times the parents were excluded, while at other times it was the young adult who was excluded. The time of diagnosis is one where a great deal of information is provided to the patient, and it is widely recognized that this may result in information overload. Healthcare providers may use medical terminology that is too technical for lay individuals to understand, not unlike when information is given to older adults with cancer. However, confusion may result when the young adult has to pass on this information to parents who were not present at the appointment.

Treatment Decisions

By law, anyone age 18 and older is allowed to make decisions about health care and treatment of disease autonomously. This can cause problems in families where the parents are uncomfortable with the decisions that the young adult makes. Grinyer and Thomas (2001) described the actions of a young man diagnosed with terminal lymphoma. He chose to travel overseas with friends instead of receiving treatment and died weeks later without ever seeing his parents again. This may be an extreme example, but conflict can arise in many different situations. For example, conflict is likely when a young adult refuses chemotherapy because he or she does not want to experience hair loss, and the parents want the young adult to have the most aggressive treatment to optimize chances of remission.

Parents often accompany their young adult child to medical appointments. Doshi et al. (2014) reported a variety of reasons why mothers attend appointments with young adult survivors. These reasons include concern for the health and well-being of the young adult, practical support, transportation, family tradition (always going with the child to appointments), general support, companionship, personal interest on the part of the mother about follow-up care, specific characteristics of the child including age (younger than 18 years old), emotional support, and a sense of parental duty. Young adults may decide to withhold information from their parents or refuse to allow them to attend medical appointments. This can be devastating to parents who want to help and support their child and feel left out and helpless.

Caring for the Young Adult With Cancer

One of the most critical challenges for parents of young adults with cancer is the need for practical support. Having to take care of the physical needs of a young adult is difficult for parents who have not had to provide that kind of care for many years. Parents of young adults with cancer may find themselves having to help their child with toileting, bathing, eating, and doing other intimate activities that hark back to the days when the young adult was a very young child or baby. The response of the young adult to this apparent regression may be to demonstrate challenging behavior (Grinyer & Thomas, 2001). This "acting out" may cause additional stress to the parents and also affect other family members, such as siblings.

Young adults with cancer face issues related to control of their body, something that is very difficult to deal with. They may choose to do things that their parents disapprove of in an attempt to have control over something. It is not unusual for young adults to get one or more tattoos or piercings; this is one way of controlling what happens to their body, but it may be upsetting to those parents who hold certain views about body art. Parental disapproval may extend to other behaviors as well, such as smoking, alcohol use, or recreational drug use. If the young adult was living independently before the cancer diagnosis, the parents may not have been aware of these activities, and if they continue when the young adult child is living at home, this may cause significant conflict.

Parents may have to control visitors to the house; for example, if the young adults are neutropenic, visitors may expose them to the risk of infection. Visitors include friends of siblings, and limitations on this can have a negative impact on the siblings who may resent this imposition on their lives and may react negatively to this disruption. The parents may find themselves isolated from their own friends because of the pressures of caregiving, which may contribute to depression and caregiver burnout. Parents also may have to control what is said in front of the young adult out of fear of causing emotional hurt or making the situation worse (Blindheim, Thorsnes, Brataas, & Dahl, 2013).

When their young adult child is hospitalized, one or both parents may choose to stay with the child. This can have consequences for the family as a whole with other children being left in the care of extended family or friends. There may be financial consequences as well, with income loss and transportation and parking costs that are not part of the household budget. Parents may feel guilty leaving children alone in the hospital even if they are old enough to take care of themselves. Parents often are concerned that something may happen to their child if no one is watching over him or her and present to advocate for the patient with hospital staff. Barling et al. (2013) described the experiences of families where the young adult was cared for in a pediatric ward and how this was challenging because the young adult had no peers to relate to. This study also reported that the parents of hospitalized young adults perceived a lack of empathy and understanding from hospital staff. Staff who are used to working with younger children may not understand the needs of young adults and may be challenged by their developmental stage and behaviors.

Grinyer (2006) found that the mothers of young adults with a life-threatening illness experience chronic, low-grade psychological and somatic symptoms that they largely ignore and regard as low priority. In this study, women hid their own healthcare needs from professionals in an attempt to prove that they were managing to cope. Many of the women were experiencing symptoms of depression or anxiety, but these were either ignored by healthcare providers or the women were offered medication that they refused, seeing it as a sign of not being able to cope. The women in this study felt that their sadness was directly related to the life-altering diagnosis of their child and should not be pathologized but rather seen as an appropriate response to a distressing situation. The women were more emotionally engaged with their sick young adult child than their male partners, and this at times resulted in tension for the couple. Grinyer (2008) noted that while mothers take on the caring role, fathers tend to be less emotionally engaged and take a more pragmatic approach. Many would question this assumption, as fathers are equally affected by their child's illness and may have been socialized to manage their emotions in a way that appears to be disengagement.

Some young adults may not respond well to the care offered by their parents. In a study of young women with breast cancer, not all the participants were happy to accept help from their parents, as this accentuated their vulnerability and helplessness. Some of the women viewed support negatively and as an intrusion into personal space (Coyne, Wollin, & Creedy, 2012).

This discussion has focused on two-parent families; the experiences of single parents are not well described in the literature. Common sense dictates that parenting a sick young adult alone is exponentially more difficult than with a supportive partner or spouse. And little has been written about the relationship of parents with the spouse or partner of the young adult with cancer and the family dynamics with the partner's parent or parents. While there is potential for support and help in these situations, there also is potential for hurt and ill feelings during the course of the illness. Parents may not like or approve of the person their young adult child has chosen to be in a relationship with. Parents also may be upset if their child chooses his or her partner over the parents to take care of him or her.

However, parents may find that caring for the young adult is rewarding and even strengthens them personally and as a family. As difficult as it is to see a loved one suffer, learning to cope and overcome adversity is reflective of personal growth. This is actualized through finding support and learning new skills, both in coping and in doing things that give strength. A life-threatening illness in the family also serves to raise consciousness about what one values in life (Blindheim et al., 2013).

Sensitive Discussions

Parents of young adults with cancer may find themselves in the position of having to talk about sensitive issues such as fertility preservation or risks to fertility from treatment. This is a topic that most parents do not have to usually discuss with their young adult children, and it can be embarrassing for both parties. Some families may be able to deal with this through the use of gentle humor, but others may find that they do not have the vocabulary to talk about this on any level. Depending on the age of the young adult, parents may be more or less involved in the discussion and subsequent decisions about fertility preservation. Costs are always involved in fertility preservation, and the parents of young adults may have to step in and offer to pay for the procedures or even take out a bank loan to cover the costs. This may cause further tension in the family, given the unknown outcomes and the potential for money to be "wasted" on a future pregnancy that might never happen.

Sons may find it very embarrassing to talk to their mother about sperm donation, and by virtue of her caregiving role, the mother may be the only parent present when a discussion about this topic is initiated by healthcare providers. In some instances, the mother may have to transport the semen specimen to the fertility clinic, engendering strong feelings of helplessness for her son and a certain amount of embarrassment for herself.

It is important that healthcare providers assess the understanding of parents and young adults with cancer about the procedures for fertility preservation. Many people do not understand that sperm cryopreservation involves masturbation, which may be against the religious practices of some families. Parents may assume that this involves a surgical procedure and may refuse on behalf of their young adult son if they are reluctant for him to undergo further invasive procedures.

Grinyer and Thomas (2001) cited the case of one mother who realized that her son had never had the experience of a sexual relationship before his illness, and so she planned on engaging the services of a prostitute. Her son was not well enough for this to occur, but this example provides evidence of the mother's involvement in a very private and sensitive part of her son's life.

Financial Issues

As has been mentioned previously in this chapter, many families experience significant financial stresses as a result of cancer in a young adult child. One of the parents may have to take a leave of absence from work or quit entirely, and the subsequent loss of income may prove to be a very real and insurmountable hardship for many years. Grinyer and Thomas (2001) included the experience of a family who had to fight for insurance benefits for their young adult son, and this fight with bureaucracy further strained their limited resources at a time when they were already overwhelmed with caregiving responsibilities. Many hidden costs also exist in treatment, including travel to and from the hospital or cancer center, the need for ambulance transfers in emergencies or for routine care if the patient cannot be transported in a car or by public transportation, and the cost of meals for parents and other family members during extended clinic visits or hospital stays. Parents may spend money on organic and other special food to entice the young adult to eat a healthy diet. And the young adult may choose to eat fast food instead, resulting in conflict and the cost of supplements being seen as wasteful.

Young adults also may spend money on things that their parents regard as unimportant and expensive, such as long-distance telephone calls to friends, Internet charges, streaming movies, online video games, or even untested treatments online.

Sibling Relationships

Illness in young adults can cause their siblings to experience a range of emotions. It is not uncommon for siblings of young adults with cancer to feel resentful, guilty, and anxious, in addition to experiencing grief. These can change with time and extend beyond the time period that the young adult is ill, irrevocably altering the family dynamics.

Siblings may resent the amount of parental time and energy given to the young adult with cancer. Younger siblings may not recognize their feelings and may act out and seek attention in negative ways in order to cause any reaction from the parents. Younger siblings in particular may worry that they too might get cancer. It is important that they understand what the cancer is and that it is not contagious. They also may worry that something they did caused the cancer—a fight or angry words, or perhaps wishing that something bad would happen to their sibling. They may carry this guilt for a long time, and it may affect other relationships in their life.

Siblings may experience high anxiety during and after the illness of the young adult family member. One study suggested that this anxiety is related to social support; if social support is lacking, the risk of the sibling experiencing anxiety is 3.5 times higher (Eilertsen, Eilegård, Steineck, Nyberg, & Kreicbergs, 2013). This study concluded that support from parents, grandparents, and other siblings was of greatest value. Siblings who shared their feelings with other family members fared better than those who kept their feelings hidden.

The death of the young adult has long-term consequences for the siblings, who may experience psychological effects such as insecurity and difficulties dealing with loss for the rest of their lives (Grinyer, 2008). In a study from Sweden, 54% of the siblings of young adults with cancer said that they had not worked through the death of their sibling. Those who had made progress in coming to terms with the loss were more likely to be in a relationship and receiving social support (Sveen, Eilegård, Steineck, & Kreicbergs, 2014). The perception that parents and neighbors did not care for them after their brother or sister died was also associated with higher anxiety in this study. If the siblings did not share their feelings with other family members after the death of the sibling, a higher risk for subsequent anxiety was found (Eilertsen et al., 2013).

These findings suggest that parents and grandparents must find a way through their own grief to support the rest of the family. This can prove challenging, and finding a balance between caring for sick young adults, their siblings, and themselves may be impossible for some families. When the parent or parents have to work, the demands may be overwhelming. The situation is further complicated when parents have to travel to the hospital, taking valuable time away from both being at home and being with the sick young adult.

Parents' Friends and Family

Caring intensively for a family member can be an isolating experience for a number of reasons. Friends and family members who have not personally experienced the demands of caring for a sick or dying relative may be unaware of the intensity of the experience and the resulting physical and emotional consequences. Friends often ask if there is something they can do or tell the parents that if they need anything, to please call. However, parents who are caring for a sick child often do not have the energy to think about the help they need or to ask for help.

Some parents find that their friends avoid them at a time when they need support the most. This may be because friends are unsure of what to say or how to offer support or because they find that witnessing the pain and suffering is too much to bear. Because the parents do not have the energy to deal with this, friendships may collapse and never be reinstated. Those friends who do offer to help may grow tired over time, and their offers of support dwindle. The up-and-down nature of the cancer trajectory may be confusing to those who have not experienced it, and so friends may not know what to say or how to act when the young adult child experiences complications after a period of wellness. The protracted nature of cancer may make supporting the parents a lengthy endeavor, and some friends may not be able to sustain their support over time.

How to Help the Parents and Family Members of the Young Adult With Cancer

Parents of young adults with cancer can fall into three categories when it comes to dealing with the cancer diagnosis: they may be hovering, helpful, or helpless.

Hovering parents are hypervigilant, may be overprotective, and may appear to not trust staff. They often infantilize the young adult patient and interfere with any attempts at autonomy. Patience and reminders that young adults are able to make some or all of the decisions for themselves are the best responses to these parents. It is also important to remember to consult the young adults first and to not be drawn in to the actions of the parents who try to subvert this.

Helpless parents are those who are unable to move beyond their own feelings of shock, sorrow, fear, and anger and who lean on the young adult patient for support. These parents need support from staff and gentle reminders when they are overtly emotional and are upsetting their child. A referral for psychosocial support may be very helpful. This will provide them with a safe place to vent their feelings without affecting the patient.

Helpful parents are those who treat their child like the young adult he or she is, ask for help when appropriate, and respect the autonomy of the patient. Some parents become helpful after a time of helplessness or hovering.

In my book for and about young adults with cancer (Katz, 2014), I offered the following potential responses to young adults in dealing with parents.

Helpless: I need you to support me (and my partner) right now. If you cannot do that, I will have to find that support elsewhere, and that may make you feel bad. This is happening to me/us and I/we don't have the energy to support you.

Hovering: I know you mean well, and probably can't help it, but I am an adult, and this is happening to me. Your response is overwhelming me right now. I know you want to protect me, but I am actually feeling stressed and pressured by your attention. Please give me some space to process what is happening.

Helpful: Thank you. (p. 170)

Some parents offer "advice," but what they really want is obedience and for the young adult to do what they say. Other family members may send articles from newspapers, magazines, and the Internet with miracle cures or other advice that is not appropriate or evidence based, or may even contradict the treatments that are available and appropriate. Young adults may be too sick, too tired, or too stressed to manage these offers of help or advice. Having periodic family meetings can help to keep everyone aware of the plans for treatment and options for support and will provide the family and young adult a safe place to communicate in a supportive and family-focused environment where myths can be dispelled and everyone hears the same information at the same time. A family meeting also can be helpful with the parents and siblings of young adult patients to help all parties understand what is going on and to hear about the effects of the illness on each other. The presence of psychosocial clinicians (e.g., a social worker or psychologist) can be very helpful at these family meetings.

It is important for young adults with cancer to know that their health information is protected by law under the Health Insurance Portability and Accountability Act of 1996. Patients can authorize the healthcare team to release health information to others through a signed document, but it is only with this authorization that the healthcare team can share information about someone age 18 or older. All young adults should have a healthcare power of attorney that designates someone to make decisions on their behalf if they cannot speak for themselves.

The need to communicate beyond the immediate family about the progress of the young adult can be overwhelming for many patients and their families. Requests for updates about response to treatment can feel like an overwhelming task that takes time away from essential self-care and family care activities. MyLifeLine (www.mylifeline.org) is a website that allows patients or family members to set up a portal where updates can be posted and then accessed by friends and extended family. These portals have a calendar that can be created to coordinate help, such as transportation, meals, or household help. Users also can create a page to collect money to help defray the costs of treatment if desired.

Conclusion

The experience of cancer extends to the immediate family and beyond. Family dynamics can be strained when parents try their best to care for the young adult and his or her siblings. Conflicts, while not inevitable, may occur and may create negative feelings that last for years. Illness in a child is a life-altering event, and some families may not be able to cope with the demands placed on them. The cancer journey presents challenges for families, as well as opportunities for growth.

References

Barling, J.A., Stevens, J., & Davis, K.M. (2013). Family members' retrospective stories of the treatment stage of an adolescent or young adult who subsequently died of cancer. *Cancer Nursing, 36*(5), E39–E48. doi:10.1097/NCC.0b013e31829dec22

Blindheim, K., Thorsnes, S.L., Brataas, H.V., & Dahl, B.M. (2013). The role of next of kin of patients with cancer: Learning to navigate unpredictable caregiving situations. *Journal of Clinical Nursing, 22,* 681–689. doi:10.1111/j.1365-2702.2012.04349.x

Coyne, E., Wollin, J., & Creedy, D.K. (2012). Exploration of the family's role and strengths after a young woman is diagnosed with breast cancer: Views of women and their families. *European Journal of Oncology Nursing, 16,* 124–130. doi:10.1016/j.ejon.2011.04.013

Doshi, K., Kazak, A.E., Hocking, M.C., Derosa, B.W., Schwartz, L.A., Hobbie, W.L., … Deatrick, J. (2014). Why mothers accompany adolescent and young adult childhood cancer survivors to follow-up clinic visits. *Journal of Pediatric Oncology Nursing, 31,* 51–57. doi:10.1177/1043454213518111

Eilertsen, M.-E.B., Eilegård, A., Steineck, G., Nyberg, T., & Kreicbergs, U. (2013). Impact of social support on bereaved siblings' anxiety: A nationwide follow-up. *Journal of Pediatric Oncology Nursing, 30,* 301–310. doi:10.1177/1043454213513838

Grinyer, A. (2006). Caring for a young adult with cancer: The impact on mothers' health. *Health and Social Care in the Community, 14,* 311–318. doi:10.1111/j.1365-2524.2006.00622.x

Grinyer, A. (2008). The impact of cancer on parents and families. In D. Kelly & F. Gibson (Eds.), *Cancer care for adolescents and young adults* (pp. 44–58). Malden, MA: Blackwell. doi:10.1002/9780470697740.ch3

Grinyer, A., & Thomas, C. (2001). Young adults with cancer: The effects of the illness on parents and families. *International Journal of Palliative Nursing, 7,* 164–170. doi:10.12968/ijpn.2001.7.4.9032

Health Insurance Portability and Accountability Act of 1996, Pub. L. No. 104-191, 110 Stat. 1936.

Katz, A. (2014). *This should not be happening: Young adults with cancer.* Pittsburgh, PA: Hygeia Media.

Sveen, J., Eilegård, A., Steineck, G., & Kreicbergs, U. (2014). They still grieve—A nationwide follow-up of young adults 2–9 years after losing a sibling to cancer. *Psycho-Oncology, 23,* 658–664. doi:10.1002/pon.3463

CHAPTER 9
Supportive Care

Introduction

It is widely accepted that providing care to young adults with cancer encompasses much more than medical care. Attention must also be paid to their psychosocial needs, and study after study points to an abundance of unmet needs in this population. These unmet needs are directly related to the developmental growth that occurs in young adulthood, as well as to the fact that this population is underserved by existing resources in adult and pediatric settings.

The unique norms, attitudes, and beliefs of young adults determine their behaviors during and after treatment and also influence the responses of this group to the stressors inherent in the cancer experience. All young adults have concerns about who they want to be, their bodies, establishing romantic relationships, separating from their parents, making goals for careers and higher education, and creating families of their own. These tasks often are challenged by the limitations of the cancer and its treatments (Zebrack & Isaacson, 2012).

This chapter will describe supportive care from the perspective of the needs of young adults, as well as the needs that go unmet. Suggestions for closing the gap between unmet and met needs will be provided, along with the existing evidence on effective interventions focused on supporting young adults.

Supportive Care Needs

Young adults with cancer have needs for factual information about their specific cancer, practical issues related to treatment and survivorship care, emotional and interpersonal issues, and existential and spiritual issues. Informational needs encompass not only cancer- and treatment-related education but also information about risks to fertility from treatment, alterations to body image, and sexuality.

Information About Cancer

Depending on the age of the young adult with cancer, the individual's parents may try to limit the extent of detail that the oncology care team provides to the individual. Older young adults are usually independent of their parents in this regard; however, it is often challenging for healthcare providers to assess what young adults have understood and synthesized from their communication with the patient and family. The amount and detail of cancer-related information desired will be different for each individual. For some, full disclosure is empowering, whereas for others, it may be distressing (Zebrack & Isaacson, 2012). In a study of young adults with brain tumors (D'Agostino & Edelstein, 2013), participants were aware that treatment was not curative but instead was focused on delaying disease progression. For them, disease-related knowledge was framed in uncertainty.

Practical Issues

Cancer treatments and side effects cause delays and disruptions to normal life events such as schooling and employment. This isolates young adults from their peers and social life and causes great suffering. Many young adults become dependent once again on their parents for financial aid, and some are also reliant on their parents for assistance with activities of daily living (e.g., bathing, food preparation) and special care such as changing dressings or flushing IV lines. The disruption caused by treatment also affects opportunities for future employment and lifetime earning capacity (Zebrack & Isaacson, 2012), and those who experience cognitive changes because of cancer or treatment may never reach their full potential as wage earners.

Emotional Issues

Distress is a common consequence of cancer and is discussed in detail in Chapter 10. Young adults with cancer experience significant distress related to the many losses that accompany the diagnosis. Young adults, unlike young children, are able to understand the severity of their illness and experience persistent distress all along the cancer trajectory (Zebrack & Isaacson, 2012). The impact of changes on appearance and the formation of self-esteem and self-image at this crucial stage of development can be crushing. Young adult survivors may look different from their peers, and this may cause embarrassment and isolation for years after the end of treatment. Body image changes and alterations to sexuality are discussed in greater detail in Chapter 5. It is important to note that maturing young adults must form a sexual identity; the physical, social, and emotional fallout from cancer can significantly affect this developmental process, and problems related to this can influence survivors for the rest of their lives.

Young adults may experience a range of worries related to the impact of the cancer on extended family and friends. They may be concerned about the financial costs of their treatment on their parents, as well as the loss of income if one or both parents have to leave work to care for them. They may worry about the disruption in their siblings' lives because of their hospitalization and the intense focus of their parents on them. It is not unusual for young adults to try to protect their parents from worry by not telling the whole truth about test results. At the same time, they may struggle to function independently of their parents' overprotectiveness.

Interpersonal Issues

Young adulthood is a time where romantic relationships are tested and established. A detailed discussion of this is found in Chapter 4. The need for close romantic and social relationships is a fundamental aspect of young adulthood, and the challenges posed by cancer can lead to a host of problems if this is not realized.

The interruptions posed by cancer treatments, frequently requiring extended hospitalizations, can severely hamper the achievement of this milestone. Family and friends are important sources of support for young adults with cancer; however, they too may be so distressed that they are not helpful. If members of the support system are not coping with what is happening, young adult patients may be isolated and feel very alone. Sometimes friends are not able to cope with the resulting physical and emotional changes and may pull away, causing further isolation. Individuals with cancer may not be able to participate in the usual social and sporting activities of their peers because of physical limitations or lack of access to traditional locations such as bars or sports clubs because of their illness, and thus miss out on shared activities. This can cause further distancing between young adults and their peer group. Having cancer is a maturing event, and some young adult survivors find that they are not interested in the same things as their peers and therefore may seek out older or more mature friendships.

However, a study comparing young adults with cancer to their healthy peers found that during the first five years after active treatment, young adults with cancer had better global and social health-related quality of life than their healthy peers (Salsman et al., 2014). Older individuals (aged 30–39 years) fared better than those in their 20s in terms of psychosocial health. This suggests that work, relationship, and financial challenges are greater for younger survivors and that older survivors perhaps have a greater ability to deal with stressors.

Existential and Spiritual Needs

Being diagnosed with a potentially or actual life-threatening disease at a young age presents a very real existential crisis. Young adulthood is not an expected time for the threat of death, and cancer at this age goes against the "normal" order of life. The uncertainty resulting from the cancer experience can be paralyzing for some but a source of personal growth and maturation for others. Jones, Parker-Raley, and Barczyk (2011) noted that some younger cancer survivors may feel that they missed out on the normal milestones because of their illness and, when treatment is over, may attempt to return to the developmental stage they were in at the time of diagnosis. This may result in risk-taking at a time when they are expected to be past that. Some young cancer survivors report that having cancer made them more reflective and changed them for the better (Jones et al., 2011). However, witnessing the decline and death of friends of the same age due to cancer can be difficult.

An interesting analysis and literature review from Canada synthesized data about supportive care needs from a study of young adults with cancer and the extant literature on the topic (Tsangaris et al., 2014). The authors identified needs in the following areas.

Information sharing and communication: Needs in this area included the need for information that reduced fear and confusion and contributed to treatment decision making and skill acquisition. The young adults wanted treatment-related information that was detailed and yet easy to understand. The literature reviewed for this study suggested that information in electronic format was preferred, but the study participants wanted written information, information from peers, online resources, and verbal communication.

Service provision: This area refers to needs related to direct care. Both the literature and the study participants agreed on the need for multidisciplinary teams including social workers, physiotherapy, and medical subspecialists. They also agreed that a trustworthy, friendly, and knowledgeable staff was important.

Social needs: Support from family, friends, and other young adults with cancer was found to be essential in both the literature and the qualitative study. The need for increased support from others with cancer was highlighted, as the experience of others going through the same challenges was seen as being very helpful.

Psychological and emotional needs: The literature reviewed for this study identified numerous needs in this area, including autonomy, feeling normal, psychological support services, spiritual support, and feeling self-conscious about the altered body. The young adults interviewed and the literature noted that counseling services were needed along with support for challenges in the areas of sexuality and establishing intimate relationships.

Of note is that among the young adults interviewed, the need for spiritual support and guidance was important.

Physical needs: Both the literature and the young adults described multiple needs for health maintenance and help with daily practical issues such as transportation, financial matters, nutrition, exercise, and relaxation. The young adults in the study reported using marijuana for pain relief and to boost appetite.

Facility needs: The young adults interviewed and the literature identified the need for a special ward or unit where young adults could be close to others of the same age and where they could access the Internet and age-appropriate entertainment. The need for privacy was highlighted, as well as better and more accessible food.

Collaboration: Participants in the young adult study noted the need for collaboration between their medical team and their school, but this need was not found in the literature.

The needs of this population are apparent, and multiple studies corroborate both the extent of their needs and the similarities across countries. With clearly defined needs established, how well are institutions and healthcare systems meeting these needs? The following section will describe the unmet needs of young adults with cancer, emphasizing that there is much room for improvement.

Unmet Needs

Many studies have been conducted to identify the unmet needs of young adults with cancer. Using both quantitative and qualitative approaches, researchers have described gaps in service provision and resources that negatively affect quality of life. It is hoped that by describing these unmet needs, healthcare providers, administrators, and policy makers will attempt to close the gaps and meet the needs. However, study after study suggests that psychosocial needs of young adults with cancer are still unmet.

The Adolescent and Young Adult Health Outcomes and Patient Experience (AYA HOPE) Study is an ongoing initiative of the National Cancer Institute to gather data from the largest cohort of young adults with cancer to date. In an article aptly titled "'Cancer Sucks,' and Other Ponderings by Adolescent and Young Adult Cancer Survivors," Zebrack et al. (2014) identified multiple factors within five domains where the needs of these young people are not being met. All participants were within two years of diagnosis.

Medical care domain: Dissatisfaction with care was expressed in relation to lack of information about drug effects, alternative and complementary therapies, and follow-up care after treatment is over. Some were unhappy about the delay in diagnosis and how they were told they had cancer. There were complaints about the location of treatment and lack of coordination within hospitals or between healthcare providers.

Side effects and symptoms domain: Many of the participants experienced multiple side effects from treatment and as a result had poorer mental health. Because they felt so ill, some were not able to go to support group meetings or to work.

Psychological-spiritual domain: Having cancer affected several areas of the participants' lives. Many struggled with feelings of distress; fear of recurrence; issues with drugs and alcohol; multiple losses including friends, jobs, and hair; and overall a significant challenge in trying to create a sense of normality in their lives.

Relationships domain: Some of the participants talked about friends and family not acknowledging their struggles or not being willing to talk about the cancer or their feelings, as well as stressful family dynamics.

Practical domain: Many of the participants were very worried about the financial burden they or their family members were incurring. Issues about health insurance, including the complexity of the system, dominated their fears. Lost employment and having to leave school was another area that caused significant stress to these young people.

In another study using the AYA HOPE cohort (Keegan et al., 2012), researchers quantified the unmet needs of young adults. More than 50% had unmet needs for information about dealing with fear of recurrence or getting another cancer, treatment for cancer, long-term effects of treatment, and complementary and alternative treatments. Furthermore, 25%–50% had unmet information needs about healthy lifestyles, fertility, cancer risk of family members, and financial support. Nearly one-third of participants wanted to see a mental health professional, and half of these reported this as unmet. Older participants (30–39 years) were more likely than younger participants to report unmet needs. Males and non-White participants also had a greater number of unmet needs. Those who were in active treatment at the time of the study had fewer unmet needs, suggesting that the support provided during treatment met their needs for the most part and that the gaps existed in follow-up care.

In a study from Australia (Patterson, Millar, Desille, & McDonald, 2012), some different needs emerged. This small (N = 14) qualitative study identified unmet needs in the following domains: information, health care, activities of daily living, support, identity renegotiation, and distress. Of note, the participants struggled with creating a new identity for themselves in the areas of getting back on track with normal life as a young adult, resuming the developmental tasks of this stage of life, and transitioning to young adulthood after the interruption of cancer. Much of their stress was related to guilt about what their cancer had done to their families, survivor guilt, and guilt about not getting better. Another Australian study (Hall et al.,

2012) identified unmet needs related to sexuality, understanding of the healthcare system, and uncertainty about the future.

In yet another study from the AYA HOPE cohort (Smith et al., 2013), one-third of participants reported at least one unmet service need. Financial (16%), mental health (15%), and support group (14%) needs were the most commonly cited. Those who reported that they needed mental health services were more likely to report worse quality of life. This also was associated with worse fatigue, worse emotional and social functioning, and challenges at work or school. The authors of this study pointed out that the United States has a shortage of mental health workers for this population and that the demand for these professionals will increase with the Patient Protection and Affordable Care Act mandating mental health services as part of the basic medical insurance package.

The Cancer Needs Questionnaire–Young People from Australia is a 70-item instrument that measures the degree of need (none to very high) for young adults with cancer in six domains (see Figure 9-1).

How to Help the Young Adult With Cancer

The first step in meeting the supportive care needs of young adults is recognition of this population as unique with specific developmental milestone challenges. These milestones are
- Accepting personal responsibility
- Deciding on values and beliefs
- Establishing a relationship with parents that is based on equality
- Becoming financially independent.

Cancer affects each of these key milestones, and the consequences of this may be a prolonged transition to adulthood and young adults being unable to cope and requiring ongoing supervision and care. Healthcare providers can help to mitigate the effects of the cancer on development (Patterson et al., 2012). First, healthcare providers should encourage young adults to speak for themselves and should make them the focus of communication about healthcare choices and decisions. Young adult patients should also be allowed to make choices as much as possible in the daily activities of the inpatient unit (e.g., meal plans, bedtime). Also, healthcare providers can promote independence in decision making and exploration of why young adults choose what they do wherever possible in decision making. This will allow for development of values and beliefs even within the limited confines of the structured environment of cancer care. Young adults must separate from parents to gain autonomy. Healthcare providers should pay attention to the relationship of young adults with their parents and make suggestions as appropriate when the parents

---

Figure 9-1. Cancer Needs Questionnaire—Young People

CANCER NEEDS QUESTIONNAIRE
YOUNG PEOPLE

THE UNIVERSITY OF
NEWCASTLE
AUSTRALIA

We are trying to find better ways to help adolescents and young adults who have had cancer.

To do this we are asking young people about the **physical, psychological, and social needs** that they may have had since their cancer diagnosis.

For each question, please choose the answer that **best describes** your level of need. There are five choices:

No Need	All my needs were met for this issue or this was not a problem for me.
Low Need	I needed a low amount of help with this problem but was not able to get it.
Moderate Need	I needed a moderate amount of help with this problem but was not able to get it.
High Need	I needed a high amount of help with this problem but was not able to get it.
Very High Need	I needed a very high amount of help with this problem but was not able to get it.

There are no right or wrong answers. The survey will take around 10 minutes to complete. Your answers will remain strictly confidential.

The following questions ask about any needs you may have had at any time since your cancer diagnosis.

1. Treatment Environment and Care

I had the following needs...

BEFORE TREATMENT

	Cancer treatment staff telling me:	No Need	Low Need	Moderate Need	High Need	Very High Need
1	about my diagnosis	O	O	O	O	O
2	what might happen during treatment	O	O	O	O	O

(Continued on next page)

Figure 9-1. Cancer Needs Questionnaire—Young People *(Continued)*

3	whether I had the option to decline treatment	○	○	○	○	○
4	about the short term side-effects of treatment	○	○	○	○	○
5	about the long term side-effects of treatment	○	○	○	○	○
6	my chances of a full recovery	○	○	○	○	○
7	what would happen when treatment finished	○	○	○	○	○
8	whether I would be able to have children	○	○	○	○	○

DURING TREATMENT

Cancer treatment staff telling me:	No Need	Low Need	Moderate Need	High Need	Very High Need
9	whether my treatment was working	○	○	○	○	○
10	my test results as soon as possible	○	○	○	○	○
11	the way I felt was normal	○	○	○	○	○

Being able to have:	No Need	Low Need	Moderate Need	High Need	Very High Need
12	time to myself	○	○	○	○	○

AFTER TREATMENT

Cancer treatment staff telling me:	No Need	Low Need	Moderate Need	High Need	Very High Need
13	how to manage my medication	○	○	○	○	○
14	what I could do to stay healthy	○	○	○	○	○
15	what to do if I noticed a particular side-effect	○	○	○	○	○

(Continued on next page)

Figure 9-1. Cancer Needs Questionnaire—Young People *(Continued)*

THROUGHOUT TREATMENT

Having cancer treatment staff who:		No Need	Low Need	Moderate Need	High Need	Very High Need
16	listened to my concerns	O	O	O	O	O
17	treated me as an individual	O	O	O	O	O
18	were respectful	O	O	O	O	O
19	were approachable	O	O	O	O	O
20	were friendly	O	O	O	O	O
21	could have a laugh with me	O	O	O	O	O
22	explained what they were doing	O	O	O	O	O
23	spoke to me in a way that I could understand	O	O	O	O	O
24	let me talk about my feelings	O	O	O	O	O
25	let me ask questions	O	O	O	O	O
26	let me make decisions about my treatment	O	O	O	O	O
27	talked to me in private, without my family	O	O	O	O	O

AT THE CANCER TREATMENT CENTRE

Being able to have:		No Need	Low Need	Moderate Need	High Need	Very High Need
28	privacy	O	O	O	O	O
29	pleasant surroundings	O	O	O	O	O
30	good food	O	O	O	O	O
31	a choice of cancer specialists	O	O	O	O	O
32	the same cancer treatment staff throughout treatment	O	O	O	O	O
33	a choice of times for appointments	O	O	O	O	O

(Continued on next page)

Figure 9-1. Cancer Needs Questionnaire—Young People *(Continued)*

2. Education

<u>Since my cancer diagnosis</u>, I have had problems enrolling at: *(please choose as many as apply)*

S1	○ school ○ TAFE ○ university/college ○ other place of study *(please write)* _____ ○ none of the above

<u>Since my cancer diagnosis</u>, I have attended: *(please choose as many as apply)*

S2	○ school ○ TAFE ○ university/college ○ other place of study *(please write)* _____ ○ none of the above *(go to Question S3)*

I had the following needs...

WHEN STUDYING

Being able to:	No Need	Low Need	Moderate Need	High Need	Very High Need
34 attend classes	○	○	○	○	○
35 get extensions/special consideration	○	○	○	○	○
36 get guidance about study options or future career paths	○	○	○	○	○

3. Work

<u>Since my cancer diagnosis</u>, I have had problems finding work: *(please choose as many as apply)*

S3	○ full-time ○ part-time/casual ○ unpaid voluntary work ○ other type of work *(please write)* _____ ○ none of the above

(Continued on next page)

Figure 9-1. Cancer Needs Questionnaire—Young People *(Continued)*

<u>Since my cancer diagnosis,</u> **I have been employed:** *(please choose as many as apply)*

S4	O full-time O part-time/casual O unpaid voluntary work O other type of work *(please write)* _____ O none of the above *(go to Question 40)*

I had the following needs...

WHEN EMPLOYED

Knowing:		No Need	Low Need	Moderate Need	High Need	Very High Need
37	how much work I would miss	O	O	O	O	O
38	how to ask managers/co-workers for support	O	O	O	O	O
39	that managers/co-workers had support to help them cope with my situation	O	O	O	O	O

4. Information and Activities

I had the following needs...

DURING TREATMENT

Being able to:		No Need	Low Need	Moderate Need	High Need	Very High Need
40	spend time with people my own age	O	O	O	O	O
41	talk to people my age who had been through a similar experience	O	O	O	O	O

(Continued on next page)

Figure 9-1. Cancer Needs Questionnaire—Young People *(Continued)*

AT THE CANCER TREATMENT CENTRE

Being able to have:	No Need	Low Need	Moderate Need	High Need	Very High Need
42 leisure spaces and activities	O	O	O	O	O

SINCE MY CANCER DIAGNOSIS

Finding information that:	No Need	Low Need	Moderate Need	High Need	Very High Need
43 was specifically designed for me	O	O	O	O	O
44 described relaxation techniques	O	O	O	O	O

The next group of questions ask about any needs you may have had **in the last month.** *We realise that your needs may have changed during different stages of your cancer experience. Please only tell us about needs you have had in the last month. If you have not had any needs in the last month, please select 'No Need'.*

5. Feelings and Relationships

I had the following needs...

IN THE LAST MONTH

Feeling:	No Need	Low Need	Moderate Need	High Need	Very High Need
45 frustrated	O	O	O	O	O
46 anxious or nervous	O	O	O	O	O

IN THE LAST MONTH

Worrying about:	No Need	Low Need	Moderate Need	High Need	Very High Need
47 my cancer spreading	O	O	O	O	O
48 my cancer returning	O	O	O	O	O

(Continued on next page)

Figure 9-1. Cancer Needs Questionnaire—Young People *(Continued)*

49	whether my cancer treatment has worked	O	O	O	O	O
50	having cancer treatment	O	O	O	O	O
51	how my family is coping	O	O	O	O	O

IN THE LAST MONTH

Finding:	No Need	Low Need	Moderate Need	High Need	Very High Need
52 inner strength	O	O	O	O	O

IN THE LAST MONTH

Being able to:	No Need	Low Need	Moderate Need	High Need	Very High Need
53 accept my diagnosis	O	O	O	O	O
54 be independent	O	O	O	O	O

S5	**Do you have:** *(please choose as many as apply)* O a spouse/partner or boyfriend/girlfriend *(please answer Question 55)* O sibling/s or step-brothers/sisters *(please answer Questions 56–58)* O none of the above *(go to Question 59)*

I had the following needs...

IN THE LAST MONTH

Coping with:	No Need	Low Need	Moderate Need	High Need	Very High Need
55 changes in my relationship with my partner	O	O	O	O	O

IN THE LAST MONTH

Coping with:	No Need	Low Need	Moderate Need	High Need	Very High Need
56 changes in my relationships with my sibling/s	O	O	O	O	O

(Continued on next page)

Figure 9-1. Cancer Needs Questionnaire—Young People *(Continued)*

IN THE LAST MONTH

Knowing how to:	No Need	Low Need	Moderate Need	High Need	Very High Need
57	ask my sibling/s for support	O	O	O	O	O
58	give support to my sibling/s	O	O	O	O	O

6. Daily Life

I had the following needs…

IN THE LAST MONTH

Being able to:	No Need	Low Need	Moderate Need	High Need	Very High Need
59	make plans or think about the future	O	O	O	O	O

IN THE LAST MONTH

Coping with:	No Need	Low Need	Moderate Need	High Need	Very High Need
60	changes in my physical ability	O	O	O	O	O
61	changes in my appearance	O	O	O	O	O
62	not being able to do the same things as other people my age	O	O	O	O	O
63	my parent/s being overprotective	O	O	O	O	O

IN THE LAST MONTH

Managing:	No Need	Low Need	Moderate Need	High Need	Very High Need
64	pain	O	O	O	O	O
65	medication	O	O	O	O	O

(Continued on next page)

	Figure 9-1. Cancer Needs Questionnaire—Young People *(Continued)*					
66	physical side effects of treat-ment	O	O	O	O	O
67	feeling tired	O	O	O	O	O
68	loss of mobility	O	O	O	O	O
69	to take part in social activities	O	O	O	O	O
70	to travel to social events	O	O	O	O	O
	YOU HAVE NOW COMPLETED THE SURVEY **THANK YOU FOR YOUR TIME AND HELP**					
	TAFE—NSW Technical and Further Education Commission (New South Wales, Australia) *Note.* Figure courtesy of the University of Newcastle, Australia. Used with permission.					

appear to be overprotective or when the young adults defer to their parents for decisions that they should and could make for themselves. Including friends and other family members is important when promoting social networks. Finally, healthcare providers should work with schools, colleges, and employers to minimize interruption of patients' education and career, thereby protecting the young adults in their goal to achieve financial independence.

Zebrack and Isaacson (2012) posited that young adults should be treated by medical and psychosocial clinicians with expertise in this population. This is important both for appropriate treatment of the cancer, given that some young adults should be treated with pediatric protocols for certain cancers (see Chapter 3), as well as for age- and developmental stage–appropriate psychosocial care. They suggested that young adults and their parents should be encouraged to and supported in sharing their feelings and concerns about the cancer, as well as their hopes for the future; this is extremely sensitive and should be addressed by clinicians who have experience in working with families.

The importance of peer support is critical. Friendships with healthy peers should be encouraged and supported, which may mean adapting the usual routine of inpatient units to allow for late-night visits or facilitating Internet access in the hospital or clinic setting. Connecting young adults with others who have been through the cancer experience is vital; however, it also is important to support these young adults to mitigate any harmful effects of reliving their own negative experiences in the process of providing peer support.

Communication with healthcare providers is a key aspect of supportive care, and it is very important to young adults that the care team speaks to them honestly and directly. They can detect a patronizing or condescending attitude very quickly, and this will erode any hope of trust being established and will affect adherence to treatment. It also is suggested that healthcare providers prepare young adult survivors for the challenges that lie ahead in social situations, such as insensitive remarks about their appearance, discrimination if they are visibly disabled, and even stigmatization by friends and family members (Zebrack, Chesler, & Kaplan, 2010).

Interventions for the Provision of Supportive Care

A study conducted with 20 young adult survivors (5 men and 15 women) highlighted what these survivors saw as important programs to address supportive care needs (Rabin, Simpson, Morrow, & Pinto, 2011). They identified the following interventions as important components of programs.

- Physical activity: Benefits of this were described as improved mental health, relaxation, prevention of weight loss, recovery from treatment, and increased physical strength.
- Relaxation: Different types of activities to promote relaxation (yoga, meditation, mindfulness, deep breathing, massage, Reiki, and laughter) were described as ways to reduce stress, facilitate the mind-body connection, reduce the severity of symptoms such as pain, and promote the processing of emotions.
- Emotional support: The young adults found one-on-one peer support and support groups to be helpful in dealing with the emotional side effects of having cancer, including depression, anxiety, and self-blame. Survivors felt that peer support was far superior to support from family and friends, who could not be objective and did not know what it was like for the survivor.
- Nutrition/weight management: Information about nutrition was seen as an important part of a healthy lifestyle after cancer.
- Information: Survivors detailed a range of topics that they deemed important, including insurance, fertility, and talking to others about having cancer.
- Similarity in groups: Participants felt it was important that supportive care programs be provided in groups where survivors were similar in terms of age, sex, and cancer and treatment type.

Some programs have been evaluated and were found to be uniformly positive. A four-day program focusing on advocacy skills acquisition at Camp Mak-A-Dream was shown to help participants deal with multiple issues, such as coping with uncertainty after treatment is over, body image concerns, worries about sexuality, fertility, and options for careers (Zebrack, Oeffinger, Hou, & Kaplan, 2006). Another program, a one-day conference, was shown to increase young adult survivors' knowledge about the need for a healthy diet, stress reduction, and exercise as part of survivorship, as well as increased knowledge about late effects of cancer treatment (Sadak, Connor, & DeLuca, 2013).

An interesting online cognitive-behavioral therapy intervention is being tested in Australia (Sansom-Daly et al., 2012). This randomized controlled trial will determine the feasibility and efficacy of an intervention called "ReCaPTure LiFe–AYA" (Resilience and Coping skills for young People and their families To Live well Following cancer–Adolescent and Young Adult version) that is provided online over six weeks in 90-minute group sessions. The content of the sessions includes

- Psychoeducation (learning positive coping skills and normalizing concerns and fears)
- Healthy living (incorporating structure and positive events into life as a survivor)
- Appraisal (dealing with body changes, friendships, self-esteem, and negative thoughts)
- Acceptance (dealing with fear of recurrence and long-term effects)
- Social support (reconnecting with friends and negotiating difficult situations after cancer).

Organizations Providing Supportive Care

In recognition of the unique needs of this population, a number of organizations have been founded to address these needs. They offer interesting and innovative approaches to providing supportive care to young adults; many focus on peer support as a central aspect.

- Camp Mak-A-Dream (for young adults and teens): www.campdream.org
- First Descents (ages 18–39): www.firstdescents.org
- Living Beyond Breast Cancer (initiatives specific to young women with breast cancer): www.lbbc.org
- Next Step (for those up to 40 years of age with various life-threatening illnesses): www.nextstepnet.org
- Prepare to Live (ages 18–40): www.preparetolive.org
- Stupid Cancer (ages 15–39): www.stupidcancer.org
- Teen Impact (ages 13–30+): www.teenimpactprogram.com
- Teens Living With Cancer (ages 13–22): www.teenslivingwithcancer.org
- Ulman Cancer Fund for Young Adults (ages 15–35): www.ulmanfund.org
- Vital Options International (ages 18–40): www.vitaloptions.org
- Young Adult Cancer Canada (ages 15–39): www.youngadultcancer.ca
- Young Survival Coalition (women ages 15–40 with breast cancer): www.youngsurvival.org

Conclusion

This chapter has highlighted the supportive care needs of young adults with cancer, as well as the ways in which these needs are not being met. Gaps exist in all domains of functioning, and few tested interventions or services are available to fulfill these unmet needs. Despite the resilience of youth, ongoing suffering results from the gaps in service provision and lack of effective interventions.

References

D'Agostino, N.M., & Edelstein, K. (2013). Psychosocial challenges and resource needs of young adult cancer survivors: Implications for program development. *Journal of Psychosocial Oncology, 31,* 585–600. doi:10.1080/07347332.2013.835018

Hall, A.E., Boyes, A.W., Bowman, J., Walsh, R.A., James, E.L., & Girgis, A. (2012). Young adult cancer survivors' psychosocial well-being: A cross-sectional study assessing quality of life, unmet needs, and health behaviors. *Supportive Care in Cancer, 20,* 1333–1341. doi:10.1007/s00520-011-1221-x

Jones, B.L., Parker-Raley, J., & Barczyk, A. (2011). Adolescent cancer survivors: Identity paradox and the need to belong. *Qualitative Health Research, 21,* 1033–1040. doi:10.1177/1049732311404029

Keegan, T.H.M., Lichtensztajn, D.Y., Kato, I., Kent, E.E., Wu, X.-C., West, M.M., ... AYA HOPE Study Collaborative Group. (2012). Unmet adolescent and young adult cancer survivors information and service needs: A population-based cancer registry study. *Journal of Cancer Survivorship, 6,* 239–250. doi:10.1007/s11764-012-0219-9

Patient Protection and Affordable Care Act, Pub. L. No. 111-148, 124 Stat. 119 (2010).

Patterson, P., Millar, B., Desille, N., & McDonald, F. (2012). The unmet needs of emerging adults with a cancer diagnosis: A qualitative study. *Cancer Nursing, 35,* E32–E40. doi:10.1097/NCC.0b013e31822d9105

Rabin, C., Simpson, N., Morrow, K., & Pinto, B. (2011). Behavioral and psychosocial program needs of young adult cancer survivors. *Qualitative Health Research, 21,* 796–806. doi:10.1177/1049732310380060

Sadak, K.T., Connor, C., & DeLuca, H. (2013). Innovative educational approaches to engage and empower the adolescent and young adult childhood cancer survivor. *Pediatric Blood and Cancer, 60,* 1919–1921. doi:10.1002/pbc.24635

Salsman, J.M., Garcia, S.F., Yanez, B., Sanford, S.D., Snyder, M.A., & Victorson, D. (2014). Physical, emotional, and social health differences between posttreatment young adults with cancer and matched healthy controls. *Cancer, 120,* 2247–2254. doi:10.1002/cncr.28739

Sansom-Daly, U.M., Wakefield, C.E., Bryant, R.A., Butow, P., Sawyer, S., Patterson, P., ... Cohn, R.J. (2012). Online group-based cognitive-behavioural therapy for adolescents and young adults after cancer treatment: A multicenter randomised controlled trial of Recapture Life-AYA. *BMC Cancer, 12,* 339. doi:10.1186/1471-2407-12-339

Smith, A.W., Parsons, H.M., Kent, E.E., Bellizzi, K., Zebrack, B.J., Keel, G., ... AYA HOPE Study Collaborative Group. (2013). Unmet support service needs and health-related quality of life among adolescents and young adults with cancer: The AYA HOPE study. *Frontiers in Oncology, 3,* 75. doi:10.3389/fonc.2013.00075

Tsangaris, E., Johnson, J., Taylor, R., Fern, L., Bryant-Lukosius, D., Barr, R., ... Klassen, A. (2014). Identifying the supportive care needs of adolescent and young adult survivors of cancer: A qualitative analysis and systematic literature review. *Supportive Care in Cancer, 22,* 947–959. doi:10.1007/s00520-013-2053-7

Zebrack, B., Chesler, M.A., & Kaplan, S. (2010). To foster healing among adolescents and young adults with cancer: What helps? What hurts? *Supportive Care in Cancer, 18,* 131–135. doi:10.1007/s00520-009-0719-y

Zebrack, B., & Isaacson, S. (2012). Psychosocial care of adolescent and young adult patients with cancer and survivors. *Journal of Clinical Oncology, 30,* 1221–1226. doi:10.1200/JCO.2011.39.5467

Zebrack, B., Kent, E.E., Keegan, T.H.M., Kato, I., Smith, A.W., & AYA HOPE Study Collaborative Group. (2014). "Cancer sucks," and other ponderings by adolescent and young adult cancer survivors. *Journal of Psychosocial Oncology, 32,* 1–15. doi:10.1080/07347332.2013.855959

Zebrack, B.J., Oeffinger, K.C., Hou, P., & Kaplan, S. (2006). Advocacy skills training for young adult cancer survivors: The Young Adult Survivors Conference at Camp Mak-A-Dream. *Supportive Care in Cancer, 14,* 779–782. doi:10.1007/s00520-005-0906-4

CHAPTER 10
Distress

Introduction

A diagnosis of cancer represents a life-altering and life-threatening event, particularly in young adults. The cancer journey encompasses many stressors, including the shock of diagnosis, repeated invasive procedures, treatment side effects that may persist for many years, the need for follow-up for an extended time (usually years), and an altered life plan, including changes in career or occupation, family planning, and perhaps even premature death. These stressors commonly lead to the experience of distress, and in some instances, to a severe form of distress, post-traumatic stress symptoms or disorder. It is possible, however, to overcome the stress and distress and experience post-traumatic growth, a transcendent experience linked to finding meaning in the experience.

Distress in Cancer

The National Comprehensive Cancer Network® (NCCN®) defines distress in cancer as a multifactorial unpleasant emotional experience that may interfere with the person's ability to cope effectively with cancer symptoms and treatment (NCCN, 2014). Distress is seen as occurring on a continuum from normal feelings of sadness and fear to disabling situations such as depression, panic, social isolation, and existential crisis.

As with most psychosocial topics, this is an understudied area in young adults. However, it is theorized that because young adults are at a critical life stage, they may be more distressed than older adults. In a concept analysis of the experience of people with acute leukemia, Albrecht and Rosenzweig (2014) proposed that the causes of distress include age, gender, and other demographic factors, personality characteristics, values, life experience, coping, resilience, and self-esteem, as well as social support. Disease factors play a role too; stage of disease, length of stay in the hospital or pro-tracted treatment, and communication with the healthcare team all influ-ence the occurrence of distress. They concluded that the consequences of distress include quality-of-life effects in all domains of functioning (physical, psychological, social, and spiritual), as well as health outcomes, including adherence to treatment.

Kwak et al. (2013b) studied 215 young adult patients at 4, 6, and 12 months after diagnosis. Levels of distress were high at the time of diagnosis, decreased at the 6-month mark, and then increased again at the 12-month mark when transition from active treatment occurred. They found that not being in school or employed contributed to distress. In another analysis of the same cohort (Zebrack et al., 2014), 35% of the sample reported clini-cally significant distress at least once during the study period, and 27% were distressed at the one-year point. Participants reported multiple unmet needs for support; 57% reported needs for information, 41% for counseling, and 39% for practical support. The authors concluded that young adults may resist asking for help because of the stigma associated with mental health services or because they did not want to be seen as different from their peers. However, 25% of the sample demonstrated a resilient coping style. These survivors tended to be older and remained in school or were employed.

In another study of 322 young adults with cancer (Yanez, Garcia, Victor-son, & Salsman, 2013), distress was highest between 13 and 24 months after diagnosis. Interruption to work or school attendance were factors associ-ated with increased distress. This time period is described as the reentry phase wherein contact with the medical system decreases. It also is a time when life is supposed to return to "normal" and long-term and late effects of treatment become apparent. The authors suggested that when expectations about life after cancer are not met and survivors continue to experience problems related to treatment, distress might be exacerbated. For those sur-vivors who do not go back to work or attend school, distress may continue up to and possibly beyond the five-year mark.

Distress can lead to tragic consequences. In a study from Iceland, young adults with cancer were assessed as being at high risk for suicide, particu-larly during the first year after diagnosis. Lu et al. (2013) compared com-pleted suicides versus expected suicides in the population. The relative risk during the first year after diagnosis was 2.5 (95% confidence interval [CI] [1.7, 3.5]) and 1.5 (95% CI [1.2, 1.8]) after that. Suicide risk was increased among those diagnosed with a potentially lethal cancer (excluding thyroid cancer, testicular cancer, and melanoma).

Not being prepared for lingering side effects can be a source of dis-tress and may result in self-doubt and the survivors questioning whether they made the right decisions related to treatment (Rosedale & Fu, 2010). For those who are caring for children, the limitations posed by treatment side effects may be particularly distressing. This is supported by the results of a study of women with breast or gynecologic cancer (Gómez-Campelo, Bragado-Álvarez, & Hernández-Lloreda, 2014). Younger women were more distressed than their older peers, and those who had not yet completed childbearing were also more distressed.

In a review of coping in young cancer survivors (Rosen, Rodriguez-Wallberg, & Rosenzweig, 2009), coping styles were seen to mitigate distress. Those with an internal locus of control, an optimistic outlook, a tendency to minimize problems, and a tendency to reframe situations in a positive manner were likely to experience less distress. Those who use an avoidant coping style, engage in wishful thinking and self-blame, and tend to be fatalistic were seen to experience greater distress.

Siblings of young adults with cancer also can experience distress. A study of 106 siblings of individuals with cancer (McDonald, Patterson, White, Butow, & Bell, 2014) suggested that distress was higher for siblings during active treatment or after recurrence. This may reflect family dynamics such as absent parents at times of high disease acuity. Siblings may not be given information about what is happening, and so their distress may increase because of worry about what might happen. Older siblings in this study were less distressed; this may reflect their relative decreased engagement in the family as they interact with their peers or they may have fewer unmet needs because of increasing maturity.

Screening for Distress

The American College of Surgeons Commission on Cancer (2012) requires screening for distress for all patients beginning in 2015. This is an accreditation standard; therefore, all institutions and treatment centers seeking to achieve or maintain accreditation will have to show evidence of screening for distress. NCCN (2014) guidelines state that distress should be screened for at the initial visit using a valid screening tool, at appropriate intervals, and at times when change has occurred in the disease trajectory (e.g., recurrence, remission, progression). It is vital that appropriate staff members are trained to deal with any distress identified, and this should be managed according to established guidelines.

NCCN has created the Distress Thermometer as a screening tool (see Figure 10-1). The thermometer itself is an easy visual tool to indicate distress, and the accompanying problem list allows for inclusion of problems during the past week that provides additional information for healthcare providers to act on. The Distress Thermometer is a screening tool only and not a diagnostic tool; identification of patients with distress must be accompanied by further assessment of psychological status and subsequent treatment.

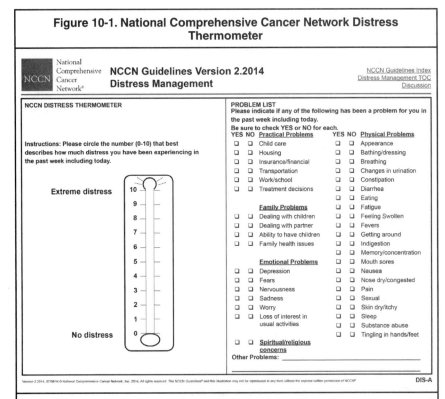

Figure 10-1. National Comprehensive Cancer Network Distress Thermometer

Patients at increased risk for distress include those with (NCCN, 2014)
- A history of substance abuse
- A psychiatric disorder
- Cognitive impairment
- Language, literacy, or physical barriers
- Severe comorbid illness
- Social issues
  - Family conflict
  - Poor social support
  - Living alone
  - Financial problems
  - Younger age

– Female sex
– Dependent children
– History of physical or sexual abuse.

The American Society of Clinical Oncology (Andersen et al., 2014) has adopted and endorsed (with minor changes) a pan-Canadian guideline for the screening, assessment, and care of distress in adults with cancer. The guideline applies to those 18 years of age and older at any time during the cancer trajectory. The recommendations are that all patients with cancer be evaluated for signs of distress (anxiety and depression) at periodic times using validated measures that have reportable scores and are clinically meaningful with appropriate cutoff points. Depending on the distress noted, treatment should be provided. It also is recommended that health-care providers be aware of the resources in their institutions and communities where treatment for their patients is available.

Carlson, Waller, and Mitchell (2012) recommended that before initiation of routine screening for distress, training of staff who will be doing the screening and subsequent referrals is essential. They stated that screening must be linked to follow-up care and treatment. These authors also noted that screening for distress should be accompanied by assessment of unmet needs.

A joint task force comprising the American Psychosocial Oncology Society, Association of Oncology Social Work, and Oncology Nursing Society (Pirl et al., 2014) developed recommendations for screening programs in cancer centers in response to the requirements of the American College of Surgeons. They identified a number of screening tools, such as the NCCN Distress Thermometer, and suggested a protocol for screening that included

- A staff member administers the screening tool, collects the completed tool, and ensures that the completed screening tool is reviewed by a qualified staff person.
- A clinician (or team of clinicians) reviews the completed screening tools and decides which patients require further assessment.
- A clinician (or team of clinicians) contacts the patients deemed to be experiencing distress for further follow-up and management.

The purpose of follow-up is to explore the nature of the distress being experienced by patients and determine what actions should follow. The task force recommended that when distress is identified, the NCCN guidelines for management of distress should be followed (Pirl et al., 2014). Tavernier, Beck, and Dudley (2013) suggested that having the Distress Thermometer integrated into the electronic health record as well as allowing patients to complete the tool electronically would be beneficial to adoption of the screening recommendations.

Social workers are the most likely members of the team who would address distress-related concerns in patients. Findings of a study of the experiences of oncology social workers (Oktay, Nedjat-Haiem, Davis, & Kern, 2012) revealed that social workers are concerned about being unable to meet the needs of patients when a screening program is implemented. Their concerns relate to workload and the potential for missing patients in high distress. They also were concerned about the potential for false positives and negatives of screening tools and of the refusal of some distressed patients to meet with social workers. On the other hand, these social workers saw multiple benefits to distress screening, including establishing relationships with patients, improving collaboration with other healthcare professionals, and showing the value of social work.

In another study of various oncology care providers in the United Kingdom (Absolom et al., 2011), while the responsibility for identifying patients who were distressed fell on all members of the team, nurses, particularly clinical nurse specialists, were regarded as the professionals most responsible for screening for and managing distress.

Barriers to Screening

Despite the previously cited recommendations, not all clinicians accept the idea that screening for distress is helpful. Mitchell, Lord, Slattery, Grainger, and Symonds (2012) conducted a study of 50 clinicians (chemotherapy nurses and radiographers/radiation technologists) who were asked to implement a screening program and provide feedback after each clinical encounter where the screening was used. Screening was seen as useful in only 43% of assessments, not useful in 35.9% of assessments, and neutral in the remaining 21% of assessments. More than 50% of those participating reported that screening was helpful with communication, and 37.5% believed that screening for distress was impractical for routine use. The chemotherapy nurses had greater difficulty than the radiation therapy staff in including distress screening in their initial assessments of patients. Barriers to screening included lack of time, insufficient training of staff, and low confidence in the screening. However, for those participants who were willing to screen patients, improvements in communication and the detection of psychological problems were seen as beneficial to both patients and care providers.

Other researchers have identified similar barriers. In a study of members of the Oncology Nursing Society (Tavernier et al., 2013), only 23% were very familiar with the NCCN guidelines for distress management, and just 17% reported using the Distress Thermometer with their patients. A further 13% indicated that they used some other tool, while 59% did not use any tool to assess for distress. Advanced practice nurses were perceived to be the healthcare providers who valued distress screening the most.

Tools for Screening for Distress

A number of validated tools exist for distress screening, including the previously discussed Distress Thermometer and Problem List (NCCN, 2014). This instrument is copyrighted, and approval must be received from NCCN to use it.

The Edmonton Symptom Assessment Scale (ESAS) is a tool used commonly in Canada. It has established validity and reliability and screens for nine common symptoms (pain, fatigue, nausea, depression, anxiety, drowsiness, appetite, well-being, and dyspnea). The severity of each symptom is assessed on a 0–10 scale, with 0 indicating that the symptom is absent and 10 indicating extreme severity. It usually is accompanied by the Canadian Problem Checklist that asks about 21 additional items not covered in the ESAS. The ESAS, along with guidelines for use and a link to translated versions, is available to download from www.palliative.org/tools.html, and the Canadian Problem Checklist is available in the booklet at www.partnershipagainst cancer.ca/wp-content/uploads/2.4.0.1.4.5-Guide_CJAG.pdf.

Post-Traumatic Stress

All of the stressors in the cancer journey have the potential to move individuals past the anticipated "normal" distress to a range of responses that can be classified as *post-traumatic stress symptoms* (PTSS).

PTSS may occur both acutely (at the time of diagnosis) and chronically (during treatment and beyond). These symptoms include (a) reexperiencing the event with intrusive thoughts or memories or even nightmares, (b) avoidance of thoughts, feelings, and reminders of the event, including missing appointments, and emotional numbing, and (c) hypervigilance and arousal, including repeated self-examination of the body or the area affected by cancer and sleep disturbances. Jim and Jacobsen (2008) suggested that post-traumatic stress occurs as a result of the struggle to integrate information related to the trauma with core beliefs. When this is considered in young adults with cancer, the core beliefs of immortality, invulnerability, and invincibility clash with the possibility of cancer as a life-threatening condition.

Intrusive thoughts are a common symptom of post-traumatic stress. These may be manifested as thinking about the cancer even when the person does not want to or repeatedly reliving aspects of the cancer, such as hearing the diagnosis for the first time or the images, sounds, and smells of the treatment area or hospital. This may result in a conscious effort to avoid any memories of the cancer, and survivors may use emotional numbing or avoidance as coping strategies. Hypervigilance is common as well, but the symptoms of physiologic arousal (difficulty concentrating and sleep disturbance) may be confused with side effects of treatment. The fear of recurrence may promote the need to be hypervigilant. Younger cancer survivors are thought to be more likely to experience PTSS.

A diagnosis of *post-traumatic stress disorder* (PTSD) can be made if the person experiences a traumatic event and the event causes significant distress or impairment to social interactions, ability to work, or other areas of functioning. Four distinct clusters are associated with PTSD: reexperiencing, avoidance, negative mood or cognition, and arousal. The condition has to continue for more than a month in order to be considered PTSD (American Psychiatric Association, 2013).

PTSS and PTSD have been studied minimally in young adults with cancer, even though young age has been identified as a risk factor for the development of PTSD (Abbey, Thompson, Hickish, & Heathcote, 2014). Kwak et al. (2013a) found that in a sample of 151 young adults, 44% reported moderate levels of symptoms one year after diagnosis and 3% experienced severe levels of stress. These participants may still have been under treatment at this time, as many treatment protocols are lengthy. Furthermore, 29% of the participants were at risk for a diagnosis of PTSD, suggesting persistent symptoms characteristic of prolonged treatment and distressing experiences. The researchers found that those who experienced greater side effects from treatment were, not surprisingly, at greater risk for PTSS. Moderating factors included maintaining employment or school attendance. Of note is that participants who were diagnosed with so-called good cancers with high survival rates experienced higher levels of PTSS. The conclusion reached about this seemingly counterintuitive result was that participants struggled with their fears of the future despite assurances from their oncology team that they have a "good cancer" relative to others or that they will be cured. It also was suggested that those with cancers with high cure rates may have less contact with their medical team and receive less support. An additional result of this study was that levels of PTSS stabilize in the first 6–12 months after diagnosis.

The parents of young adults with cancer also may experience PTSS. Yonemoto, Kamibeppu, Ishii, Iwata, and Tatezaki (2012) found that parents experienced higher levels than their children who had cancer. However, this was a younger population of patients (ages 7–18 at diagnosis), and parental worry may be higher the younger the child. A search of the literature related to parents of young adults did not produce any studies.

The flip side of post-traumatic stress is that of benefit-finding and, ultimately, post-traumatic growth (PTG). *Benefit-finding* is a process wherein the individual assigns a positive value to the experience and may be a precursor to PTG. This involves actively working through what has happened in order to make sense of it and find the good in the experience. Benefit-finding has been associated with PTG (Mols, Vingerhoets, Coebergh, & van de Poll-Franse, 2009).

Post-Traumatic Growth

Tedeschi and Calhoun (2004) have written extensively on the topic of PTG. They stated that growth does not occur as a result of trauma but instead from the struggle that the individual faces in living with the reality of life after a trauma; this determines the extent to which growth occurs. They see growth as a consequence of stress and noted that growth can occur while the stress is still present.

PTG is transformative and reflected in a qualitative change in social and relational functioning. Helgeson, Reynolds, and Tomich (2006) proposed that intrusive thoughts, one of the hallmarks of PTSS, are ways of working through the cancer experience and trauma, and through this work, personal growth is achieved. They further suggested that a period of contemplation is needed for growth to occur.

Jim and Jacobsen (2008) stated that PTG is reported in three domains of life, which are

- Enhanced social resources (deeper love for family and partner, improved relationships, increased time and effort invested in family and friends)
- Enhanced personal resources (better outlook on life, greater spirituality, increased compassion for others)
- Improved coping skills (acceptance of circumstances, better coping with stress).

PTG is thought to be dependent on the perceived severity of the threat as well as the fear of recurrence. Younger individuals are seen to potentially experience greater PTG because, in part, they may have more flexibility in their self-concept compared to older people whose identities are more solidified (Jim & Jacobsen, 2008).

Unlike a single traumatic event (e.g., an act of nature, sexual assault), the cancer experience encompasses multiple stressors, a future orientation (will the cancer come back?), and the possibility of some control for the individual (treatment choice). Personal growth comes from suffering and, as a result, seeing oneself and the world differently. Ultimately, personal growth leads to the formation of a new identity. This identity is created by experiencing closer relationships with others, empathy, and support for others who suffer (Sumalla, Ochoa, & Blanco, 2009). Personal growth is a process that is intentional and continuous—it does not magically appear after trauma or life-threatening illness.

This process has been studied in young adults with cancer. In research on young adult survivors of osteosarcoma (Teall, Barrera, Barr, Silva, & Greenberg, 2013), compared to normative values, survivors experienced less depression. Most of the study participants had overcome the physical changes of treatment as a result of surgery and were thriving, mostly because of the support they had received that led to personal growth. In a study of young adult survivors within six months of completing treatment (Arpa-wong, Oland, Milam, Ruccione, & Meeske, 2013), 74% of the participants reported PTG. This change was largely seen in the areas of a changed sense of self and relationships with others. Young breast cancer survivors reported an association between physical activity and personal growth (Love & Sabis-ton, 2011). The authors of this study stated that the association between per-sonal growth and physical activity was greater for individuals who were inac-tive. Stress also was associated with growth.

Personal growth can be experienced as a family system rather than just on the individual level (Berger & Weiss, 2009). The theory behind this is that in response to a severe trauma or threat, families can change, and this change leads to a higher level of functioning. The authors proposed that similar to the PTG seen in individuals (sense of self, improved rela-tionships, and altered life philosophy), the family as a system displays the emergence of family identity or legacy, enhanced relationships within members and with others in the outside world, clearer priorities, and a greater appreciation for life. PTG as a family process also may involve reso-lution of past conflicts and loss and the shared creation of meaning (King & Wynne, 2004).

How to Help the Young Adult With Cancer

Distress has been described as the sixth vital sign (Bultz, Thomas, Stew-art, & Carlson, 2007) and should be monitored routinely. A limited number of interventions to promote personal growth have been studied in young adults with cancer.

Although some survivors will spontaneously experience personal growth, interventions exist that may promote this growth and meaning-making after cancer. Love and Sabiston (2011), in their study of young women with breast cancer, theorized that the association between activity and personal growth might be because physical activity may enhance self-perception. Therefore, they concluded that physical activity could be an effective intervention for young adults after cancer treatment. In an Australian study (Dunn, Camp-bell, Penn, Dwyer, & Chambers, 2009), women with breast cancer partici-pated in a seven-day motorbike ride to raise awareness of breast cancer. The study found that many of the women were motivated to take part as a way of gaining control of their lives, as well as because of a desire for personal growth. PTG occurred for many, but not all, of the women. The peer sup-port experienced as part of the ride itself generated positive feelings for 85% of the riders, including a positive perspective shift. About 15% of the women did not experience close social connections and felt disappointed. The process of growth identified by the researchers occurred in the context of a physical challenge (the ride) in a new setting with social support from a group of peers.

Although it did not identify personal growth as an outcome, a novel trial of a therapeutic music video intervention found that aspects of growth resulted from the intervention among young adults undergoing stem cell transplantation (Robb et al., 2014). The intervention comprised a three-week, six-session process of creating a music video, including writing songs and developing a video. The intervention took place while the participants were in the hospital. In comparison with a control group, program participants improved courageous coping immediately after completing the video and improved social integration and family relationships measured 100 days after the transplant. They also showed signs of improved spiritual perspective and self-transcendence, both of which are hallmarks of PTG.

Conclusion

The experience of distress is universal in individuals with cancer, and although healthcare providers cannot prevent this phenomenon from occurring, screening and intervention may prevent it from progressing to a pathologic problem such as PTSD. The flip side of distress is personal growth, which presents opportunities for individuals with cancer and their family members to derive meaning from a difficult chapter in life.

References

Abbey, G., Thompson, S.B.N., Hickish, T., & Heathcote, D. (2014). A meta-analysis of prevalence rates and moderating factors for cancer-related post-traumatic stress disorder. *Psycho-Oncology*. Advance online publication. doi:10.1002/pon.3654

Absolom, K., Holch, P., Pini, S., Hill, K., Liu, A., Sharpe, M., ... Velikova, G. (2011). The detection and management of emotional distress in cancer patients: The views of health-care professionals. *Psycho-Oncology, 20*, 601–608. doi:10.1002/pon.1916

Albrecht, T.A., & Rosenzweig, M. (2014). Distress in patients with acute leukemia: A concept analysis. *Cancer Nursing, 37*, 218–226. doi:10.1097/NCC.0b013e31829193ad

American College of Surgeons Commission on Cancer. (2012). *Cancer program standards 2012: Ensuring patient-centered care* [v.1.2.1, released January 2014]. Retrieved from http://www.facs.org/cancer/coc/programstandards2012.html

American Psychiatric Association. (2013). *Diagnostic and statistical manual of mental disorders* (5th ed.). Arlington, VA: American Psychiatric Publishing.

Andersen, B.L., DeRubeis, R.J., Berman, B.S., Gruman, J., Champion, V.L., Massie, M.J., ... Rowland, J.H. (2014). Screening, assessment, and care of anxiety and depressive symptoms in adults with cancer: An American Society of Clinical Oncology guideline adaptation. *Journal of Clinical Oncology, 32*, 1605–1619. doi:10.1200/JCO.2013.52.4611

Arpawong, T.E., Oland, A., Milam, J.E., Ruccione, K., & Meeske, K.A. (2013). Post-traumatic growth among an ethnically diverse sample of adolescent and young adult cancer survivors. *Psycho-Oncology, 22,* 2235–2244. doi:10.1002/pon.3286

Berger, R., & Weiss, T. (2009). The posttraumatic growth model: An expansion to the family system. *Traumatology, 15,* 63–74. doi:10.1177/1534765608323499

Bultz, B.D., Thomas, B.C., Stewart, D.A., & Carlson, L.E. (2007). Distress—The sixth vital sign in cancer care: Implications for treating older adults undergoing chemotherapy. *Geriatrics and Aging, 10,* 647–653.

Carlson, L.E., Waller, A., & Mitchell, A.J. (2012). Screening for distress and unmet needs in patients with cancer: Review and recommendations. *Journal of Clinical Oncology, 30,* 1160–1177. doi:10.1200/JCO.2011.39.5509

Dunn, J., Campbell, M., Penn, D., Dwyer, M., & Chambers, S.K. (2009). Amazon heart: An exploration of the role of challenge events in personal growth after breast cancer. *Journal of Psychosocial Oncology, 27,* 119–135. doi:10.1080/07347330802616084

Gómez-Campelo, P., Bragado-Álvarez, C., & Hernández-Lloreda, M.J. (2014). Psychological distress in women with breast and gynecological cancer treated with radical surgery. *Psycho-Oncology, 23,* 459–466. doi:10.1002/pon.3439

Helgeson, V.S., Reynolds, K.A., & Tomich, P.L. (2006). A meta-analytic review of benefit finding and growth. *Journal of Consulting and Clinical Psychology, 74,* 797–816. doi:10.1037/0022 -006X.74.5.797

Jim, H.S.L., & Jacobsen, P.B. (2008). Posttraumatic stress and posttraumatic growth in cancer survivorship: A review. *Cancer Journal, 14,* 414–419. doi:10.1097/PPO.0b013e31818d8963

King, D.A., & Wynne, L.C. (2004). The emergence of "family integrity" in later life. *Family Process, 43,* 7–21. doi:10.1111/j.1545-5300.2004.04301003.x

Kwak, M., Zebrack, B.J., Meeske, K.A., Embry, L., Aguilar, C., Block, R., … Cole, S. (2013a). Prevalence and predictors of post-traumatic stress symptoms in adolescent and young adult cancer survivors: A 1-year follow-up study. *Psycho-Oncology, 22,* 1798–1806. doi:10.1002/pon.3217

Kwak, M., Zebrack, B.J., Meeske, K.A., Embry, L., Aguilar, C., Block, R., … Cole, S. (2013b). Trajectories of psychosocial distress in adolescent and young adult patients with cancer: A 1-year longitudinal study. *Journal of Clinical Oncology, 31,* 2160–2166. doi:10.1200/ JCO.2012.45.9222

Love, C., & Sabiston, C.M. (2011). Exploring the links between physical activity and posttraumatic growth in young adult cancer survivors. *Psycho-Oncology, 20,* 278–286. doi:10.1002/ pon.1733

Lu, D., Fall, K., Sparén, P., Ye, W., Adami, H.-O., Valdimarsdóttir, U., & Fang, F. (2013). Suicide and suicide attempt after a cancer diagnosis among young individuals. *Annals of Oncology, 24,* 3112–3117. doi:10.1093/annonc/mdt415

McDonald, F.E., Patterson, P., White, K.J., Butow, P., & Bell, M.L. (2014). Predictors of unmet needs and psychological distress in adolescent and young adult siblings of people diagnosed with cancer. *Psycho-Oncology.* Advance online publication. doi:10.1002/pon.3653

Mitchell, A.J., Lord, K., Slattery, J., Grainger, L., & Symonds, P. (2012). How feasible is implementation of distress screening by cancer clinicians in routine clinical care? *Cancer, 118,* 6260–6269. doi:10.1002/cncr.27648

Mols, F., Vingerhoets, A.J.J.M., Coebergh, J.W.W., & van de Poll-Franse, L.V. (2009). Well-being, posttraumatic growth and benefit finding in long-term breast cancer survivors. *Psychology and Health, 24,* 583–595. doi:10.1080/08870440701671362

National Comprehensive Cancer Network. (2014). *NCCN Clinical Practice Guidelines in Oncology (NCCN Guidelines®): Distress management* [v.2.2014]. Retrieved from http://www.nccn.org/ professionals/physician_gls/pdf/distress.pdf

Oktay, J.S., Nedjat-Haiem, F.R., Davis, C., & Kern, K.C. (2012). Distress screening: Experiences of oncology social workers. *Journal of Psychosocial Oncology, 30,* 652–666. doi:10.1080/07347 332.2012.721490

Pirl, W.F., Fann, J.R., Greer, J.A., Braun, I., Deshields, T., Fulcher, C., … Bardwell, W.A. (2014). Recommendations for the implementation of distress screening programs in cancer centers: Report from the American Psychosocial Oncology Society (APOS), Association of Oncology Social Work (AOSW), and Oncology Nursing Society (ONS) joint task force. *Cancer, 120,* 2946–2954. doi:10.1002/cncr.28750

Robb, S.L., Burns, D.S., Stegenga, K.A., Haut, P.R., Monahan, P.O., Meza, J., … Haase, J.E. (2014). Randomized clinical trial of therapeutic music video intervention for resilience outcomes in adolescents/young adults undergoing hematopoietic stem cell transplant: A report from the Children's Oncology Group. *Cancer, 120,* 909–917. doi:10.1002/cncr.28355

Rosedale, M., & Fu, M.R. (2010). Confronting the unexpected: Temporal, situational, and attributive dimensions of distressing symptom experience for breast cancer survivors [Online exclusive]. *Oncology Nursing Forum, 37,* E28–E33. doi:10.1188/10.ONF.E28-E33

Rosen, A., Rodriguez-Wallberg, K.A., & Rosenzweig, L. (2009). Psychosocial distress in young cancer survivors. *Seminars in Oncology Nursing, 25,* 268–277. doi:10.1016/j.soncn.2009.08.004

Sumalla, E.C., Ochoa, C., & Blanco, I. (2009). Posttraumatic growth in cancer: Reality or illusion? *Clinical Psychology Review, 29,* 24–33. doi:10.1016/j.cpr.2008.09.006

Tavernier, S.S., Beck, S.L., & Dudley, W.N. (2013). Diffusion of a distress management guideline into practice. *Psycho-Oncology, 22,* 2332–2338. doi:10.1002/pon.3295

Teall, T., Barrera, M., Barr, R., Silva, M., & Greenberg, M. (2013). Psychological resilience in adolescent and young adult survivors of lower extremity bone tumors. *Pediatric Blood and Cancer, 60,* 1223–1230. doi:10.1002/pbc.24441

Tedeschi, R.G., & Calhoun, L.G. (2004). Posttraumatic growth: Conceptual foundations and empirical evidence. *Psychological Inquiry, 15,* 1–18. doi:10.1207/s15327965pli1501_01

Yanez, B., Garcia, S.F., Victorson, D., & Salsman, J.M. (2013). Distress among young adult cancer survivors: A cohort study. *Supportive Care in Cancer, 21,* 2403–2408. doi:10.1007/s00520-013-1793-8

Yonemoto, T., Kamibeppu, K., Ishii, T., Iwata, S., & Tatezaki, S. (2012). Posttraumatic stress symptom (PTSS) and posttraumatic growth (PTG) in parents of childhood, adolescent and young adult patients with high-grade osteosarcoma. *International Journal of Clinical Oncology, 17,* 272–275. doi:10.1007/s10147-011-0286-3

Zebrack, B.J., Corbett, V., Embry, L., Aguilar, C., Meeske, K.A., Hayes-Lattin, B., … Cole, S. (2014). Psychological distress and unsatisfied need for psychosocial support in adolescent and young adult cancer patients during the first year following diagnosis. *Psycho-Oncology, 23,* 1267–1275. doi:10.1002/pon.3533

CHAPTER 11
Return to Work or School

Introduction

Going back to work or school is a sentinel event for cancer survivors and a sign that some degree of normality has been achieved. Work offers much more than just a way to make a living; it is important for self-esteem, social contacts, identity, and health insurance, and for many it provides meaning and significance to life. Going back to school has similar benefits excluding immediate financial gain, although it certainly influences future work and earnings.

Although there is a growing body of literature on return to work for older cancer survivors, very little exists that is specific to young adults, and no studies have been published on the experience of young adult cancer survivors who return to college after treatment. However, web-based resources are available to support young adults as they endeavor to make the transition to "normal" work or study after cancer.

Going Back

Return to work is mediated by a number of variables, including disease-specific and treatment-related factors. The ability to return to work is influenced by demographic, health, psychosocial, motivational, and work-related factors. The role of workplace accommodation is also important in mediating a successful return to the workplace. Returning to work has work-related, financial, and psychosocial outcomes (Mehnert, 2011).

Most young adults go back to work or school after cancer treatment is over; 72% of those who were working or studying full time before cancer went back within 15–35 months (Parsons et al., 2012). Those who quit work shortly after the diagnosis were less likely to go back to work. Furthermore, 35% of the participants in this study reported that cancer had a negative impact on their future plans.

Factors that support returning to work include the perception that accommodations in the workplace and for attending follow-up appointments will be made as required (Mehnert, 2011). The flexibility of supervisors to accommodate necessary modifications also is a positive factor (Wells et al., 2013). Being able to reduce the number of work hours may help. In one study, 26% of survivors had reduced their hours, and 90% of the sample reported that they coped well within the work environment (Torp, Nielsen, Gudbergsson, & Dahl, 2012).

Challenges

Returning to work or school is challenging, and 50% of those who returned to work or school reported problems in a study by Parsons et al. (2012). These included inability to concentrate or pay attention, memory issues, and difficulty keeping up with the demands of the job or school (Parsons et al., 2012). In a review of studies about return to work (Duijts et al., 2013), the authors identified a number of factors contributing to difficulties at work, including cognitive difficulties, coping issues, depression and anxiety, and fatigue. Physical limitations, such as not being able to lift items, also can affect survivors' ability to work.

Cancer survivors are 1.5 times more likely than their healthy peers to be unemployed (de Boer, Taskila, Ojajärvi, van Dijk, & Verbeek, 2009). Young survivors are less likely to be employed and typically work fewer hours than others their same age at two to six years after diagnosis (Moran, Short, & Hollenbeak, 2011). For those who have a recurrence or second cancer, employment outcomes are poor. Physical work, the presence of fatigue and other side effects, and perceived discrimination are additional factors that can negatively affect return to work (Mehnert, 2011).

Cancer survivors may be overly optimistic about their ability to perform in the workplace. This may be reinforced when employers have negative beliefs about how cancer affects work performance (Grunfeld, Low, & Cooper, 2010).

How to Help the Young Adult With Cancer

The Americans With Disabilities Act of 1990 protects employees in workplaces with 15 or more employees (U.S. Department of Justice, n.d.). This act requires employers to make reasonable accommodations for cancer survivors who are returning to work as long as the accommodations do not cause undue hardship on the employer. Employees cannot be fired or denied benefits because of the cancer, and the employee must be allowed to take time off for medical appointments. However, discrimination in the workplace does occur, and this is against the law. The Family and Medical Leave Act of 1993 applies to workplaces with 50 or more employees and allows an employee to take up to 12 weeks of unpaid leave during a 12-month period (U.S. Department of Labor, n.d.). This act also allows family members to take leave to care for a family member who is ill. Human resources departments should know about these acts and support the employee and employer to make the necessary adjustments to the workplace.

Healthcare providers can offer the following advice to young adults with cancer who are returning to work.

- Going back to work can be physically and emotionally exhausting. Try to take it easy in the first few weeks.
- An occupational health expert can be helpful in assessing the workplace and creating a return-to-work plan that can be shared with the employer.
- This plan should include the type of work; the number of work hours and intended increase over time; what, if any, accommodations need to be made and for how long; what information can be shared with coworkers; and when the plan should be reevaluated.

Young adults who are returning to school may find the following tips to be useful.

- Communicate with student affairs and academic advisers to review progress.
- Find out what resources exist to support students in returning to school. The school may have a disabilities department that can help make accommodations in the classroom and for taking tests, obtaining tutoring, and finding adapted housing. Educational institutions are required to provide access to individuals with disabilities (including cancer) under the Americans With Disabilities Act.
- Some cancer survivors may need to take a reduced course load and may need to miss classes for medical appointments. Students should discuss this with their academic advisers and instructors.
- Student health services may be able to provide ongoing health care for issues that are not cancer related. The healthcare team should be aware of the student's health history, prescription medications, contact information for the student's primary oncologist, and any ongoing health problems.
- Student health services also can help in negotiating accommodations in course work, test taking, and tutoring.
- Although cancer survivors do not have to disclose their cancer history to academic staff, doing so can be helpful, as they can make special arrangements, such as extending deadlines on assignments or providing the student with lecture notes.

- Joining a support group for young adults with cancer in the area can provide opportunities for support and friendships with others who know what it is like to live with cancer.
- Financial aid may be available for those returning to school after cancer. FinAid (www.finaid.org/scholarships/cancer.phtml) and the SAMFund for Young Adult Survivors of Cancer (www.thesamfund.org) have information on the topic.

The following websites may be useful for cancer survivors who are returning to work or school.

- *Cancer and Returning to Work: A Practical Guide for Cancer Patients* (Parkinson, 2014): www.cw.bc.ca/library/pdf/CancerReturningToWorkManual .pdf
- Cancer and Careers: www.cancerandcareers.org
- Cancer.Net—Returning to School After Cancer: www.cancer.net/navigating -cancer-care/young-adults/life-after-treatment/returning-school-after -cancer
- *Facing Forward: Life After Cancer Treatment*—downloadable booklet from the National Cancer Institute on coping after cancer: www.cancer.gov/ publications/patient-education/facing-forward

Conclusion

Returning to work or school is an important event in the lives of young adult cancer survivors. For many, it signifies a return to normal and an opportunity to reconnect with coworkers and friends. But despite legislated protection for most workers, some will face hardships when they return. It is important that oncology care providers support survivors and provide anticipatory guidance for this transition.

References

de Boer, A.G.E.M., Taskila, T., Ojajärvi, A., van Dijk, F.J.H., & Verbeek, J.H.A.M. (2009). Cancer survivors and unemployment: A meta-analysis and meta-regression. *JAMA, 301,* 753–762. doi:10.1001/jama.2009.187

Duijts, S.F.A., van Egmond, M.P., Spelten, E., van Muijen, P., Anema, J.R., & van der Beek, A.J. (2013). Physical and psychosocial problems in cancer survivors beyond return to work: A systematic review. *Psycho-Oncology, 23,* 481–492. doi:10.1002/pon.3467

Grunfeld, E.A., Low, E., & Cooper, A.F. (2010). Cancer survivors' and employers' perceptions of working following cancer treatment. *Occupational Medicine, 60,* 611–617. doi:10.1093/ occmed/kqq143

Mehnert, A. (2011). Employment and work-related issues in cancer survivors. *Critical Reviews in Oncology/Hematology, 77,* 109–130. doi:10.1016/j.critrevonc.2010.01.004

Moran, J.R., Short, P.F., & Hollenbeak, C. (2011). Long-term employment effects of surviving cancer. *Journal of Health Economics, 30,* 505–514. doi:10.1016/j.jhealeco.2011.02.001

Parkinson, M. (2014). *Cancer and returning to work: A practical guide for cancer patients* (2nd ed.). Retrieved from http://www.cw.bc.ca/library/pdf/CancerReturningToWorkManual .pdf

Parsons, H.M., Harlan, L.C., Lynch, C.F., Hamilton, A.S., Wu, X.-C., Kato, I., ... Keegan, T.H.M. (2012). Impact of cancer on work and education among adolescent and young adult cancer survivors. *Journal of Clinical Oncology, 30,* 2393–2400. doi:10.1200/JCO.2011.39.6333

Torp, S., Nielsen, R.A., Gudbergsson, S.B., & Dahl, A.A. (2012). Worksite adjustments and work ability among employed cancer survivors. *Supportive Care in Cancer, 20,* 2149–2156. doi:10.1007/s00520-011-1325-3

U.S. Department of Justice. (n.d.). The Americans With Disabilities Act of 1990 and revised ADA regulations implementing title II and title III. Retrieved from http://www.ada .gov/2010_regs.htm

U.S. Department of Labor. (n.d.). The Family and Medical Leave Act. Retrieved from http://www.dol.gov/whd/regs/compliance/1421.htm

Wells, M., Williams, B., Firnigl, S., Lang, H., Coyle, J., Kroll, T., & MacGillivray, S. (2013). Supporting "work-related goals" rather than "return to work" after cancer? A systematic review and meta-synthesis of 25 qualitative studies. *Psycho-Oncology, 22,* 1208–1219. doi:10.1002/pon.3148

CHAPTER 12
Recurrence, Metastatic Disease, and End of Life

Introduction

Despite the rhetoric of overcoming cancer and winning the battle against cancer, not all people with cancer will remain cancer free for the rest of their lives. This is particularly important for young adults, some of whom are diagnosed with advanced cancer because of diagnostic delay as discussed in Chapter 2. Young adults also have potentially many years of life left and may carry the risk for and fear of recurrence over many years.

This chapter will describe the current evidence on recurrence and metastatic disease in young adults as well as issues related to the end of life. This chapter also addresses the issue of fear of recurrence, an important challenge for many cancer survivors and one that is perhaps even more poignant for young survivors, whose lives are, in essence, just beginning.

Risk of Recurrence

Much of what is known about recurrence in young adults comes from studies of young women with breast cancer. Recurrence can occur locally (at the site of the original cancer) or at a distance through spread to other organs (metastatic spread). Both local recurrence and distant spread are regarded as having a poor prognosis.

Young age at diagnosis is itself a factor predicting poor survival because younger women tend to have hormone receptor–negative breast cancer and an increased risk of HER2 overexpression (Copson et al., 2013; Filleron et al., 2013). Lymph node involvement increases the risk of recurrence, which is likely to occur 6–12 months after initial treatment (Filleron et al., 2013).

Siponen, Joensuu, and Leidenius (2013) reported a 6.5% local recurrence rate in women younger than age 40. In this study, mastectomy alone was the standard treatment for women with stage I or II disease or those who had positive lymph nodes. Radiation to the affected side has lowered the recurrence rate in women younger than 35 years old treated with mastectomy alone from 15% to a mere 1% (Liukkonen, Leidenius, Saarto, & Sjöström-Mattson, 2011).

The addition of endocrine manipulation therapy (such as tamoxifen for premenopausal women) further lowers recurrence rates. For women who are premenopausal when diagnosed with estrogen receptor–positive disease and have metastases, the recommendation is to include ovarian suppression (i.e., oophorectomy or treatment with a luteinizing hormone–releasing hormone agonist) and to add an aromatase inhibitor when the woman becomes postmenopausal as a result of ovarian suppression. This can cause additional side effects that affect quality of life and removes any hope for future fertility (Tichy, Lim, & Anders, 2013).

Many cancer survivors are intensely interested in preventing recurrence. Little is known about what causes recurrence, outside of poor prognostic factors at the outset. Many people believe that stress plays a causal role in both the development and recurrence of cancer. The conclusion of a systematic review of studies on the topic was that definitive evidence linking stressors of any kind to cancer recurrence did not exist (Todd, Moskowitz, Ottati, & Feuerstein, 2014). However, the authors suggested that because some evidence has linked psychological stress to recurrence, survivors should be encouraged to maintain a "healthy" level of stress. What constitutes a healthy level of stress is not described and may be impossible to achieve given the stressful nature of cancer itself.

People who are newly diagnosed with cancer often search for a cause, in part because they want to be able to prevent recurrence in the future (Miles, Simon, & Wardle, 2010). This may also be related to an attempt to regain some control in a situation that for most people is out of their control. Some evidence supports that a healthy diet may prevent recurrence, but healthcare providers often are reluctant to talk about this lifestyle factor in addition to others such as exercise and smoking cessation. Certain lifestyle issues, such as obesity, are sensitive, and perceived taboos may deter healthcare providers from talking about something that is under personal control.

Fear of Recurrence

Fear of recurrence is experienced to some degree by almost all cancer survivors—and even their family members (Vivar, Canga, Canga, & Arantzamendi,

2009)—and is thought to be one of the most distressing aspects of cancer survival (Simard, Savard, & Ivers, 2010). Because of the impact of a cancer diagnosis and subsequent treatment on the individual, survivors often feel vulnerable and uncertain about the future. Being fearful of having to go through the experience again, but this time with real knowledge of what it is like, can be very frightening; thus, fear of recurrence is normal for most individuals. However, a proportion of cancer survivors will experience fear of recurrence that leads to behaviors that are regarded as dysfunctional. These include avoidance of health care, hypervigilance for symptoms of recurrence, and inability to plan for the future. Some survivors may exhibit signs of post-traumatic stress disorder (see Chapter 10), anxiety, and depression. Fear of recurrence may be associated with intrusive thoughts and constantly recalling memories of the cancer treatment. Survivors with a high fear of recurrence may refuse to transition to a primary care provider, preferring to remain with their oncologist as they think the oncologist will be better able to monitor for recurrence. Objective risk of recurrence does not play a protective role against feelings or behaviors; even those with low risk may experience high levels of fear that the cancer will come back, despite reassurances or evidence presented by healthcare providers, and this fear may persist for many years after diagnosis (Thewes et al., 2012). Triggers for exacerbation of fear include hearing about someone else with cancer, going for follow-up care, or seeing media reports about cancer (Gil et al., 2004).

In a systematic analysis of this phenomenon in the literature, Crist and Grunfeld (2013) found that the most consistent factor in the development of this fear was young age. Other factors identified were the presence of physical symptoms, treatment type, low optimism, family stressors, and fewer significant others.

Young adults with cancer may be especially vulnerable to the development of high fear of recurrence because of psychosocial factors such as living away from family, leading to less social support; being single; and experiencing stress related to college or employment factors. Having young children is an independent predictor of fear of recurrence (Steele, Haigh, Knowles, & Mckean, 2007). In a study of young women with breast cancer, Thewes et al. (2012) reported that 70% of their sample of more than 200 women scored in the clinical range of having fear of recurrence using the Fear of Cancer Recurrence Inventory (FCRI). The women who scored high on this measure also were more likely to examine their breasts frequently, attended support groups or counseling, and made more unscheduled visits to healthcare providers. An interesting finding of this study was that although women with clinical levels of fear of recurrence examined themselves more frequently, they were less likely to adhere to the recommended medical surveillance for breast cancer, such as mammography and clinical breast examinations.

How to Help the Young Adult With Cancer

Healthcare providers should explore their patients' beliefs about recurrence in order to dispel myths and encourage effective coping. Some evidence supports that reducing stress can improve quality of life and emotional well-being. Cognitive-behavioral therapy has been shown to be effective in reducing anxiety (Osborn, Demoncada, & Feuerstein, 2006), and mindfulness-based stress reduction and yoga also have been shown to be effective in stress reduction in cancer survivors (Bower, Woolery, Sternlieb, & Garet, 2005).

Despite high levels of fear of recurrence in cancer survivors, especially those who are younger, no consensus exists on the management of this phenomenon. No clinically useful assessment tool is available that can be used as a screening instrument in busy clinics. The FCRI contains 42 items; a validated shorter tool is needed for use by oncology care providers (Thewes et al., 2012).

In a study of how fear of recurrence is managed by medical and psychosocial clinicians (Thewes et al., 2014), the authors recognized that this is a challenging phenomenon to deal with in the clinical setting. Just 21% of medical and nursing staff reported referring patients with symptoms of fear of recurrence for support. There was lack of consensus among psychosocial clinicians on how to treat this, with some using acceptance and commitment therapy while others favored cognitive-behavioral therapy. Others used psychoeducation, relaxation techniques, meditation, solution-focused therapy, or supportive therapy. These interventions have not been tested widely for use with survivors who are experiencing high levels of fear. In addition, these interventions are not widely used in practice, and medical and nursing staff may not know about them, thus limiting referrals to psychosocial clinicians. Oncology care providers should maintain an up-to-date list of psychosocial clinicians (social workers, psychologists, etc.) who they can refer to, preferably those with experience in supporting young adults with cancer. A list of support groups, both face-to-face and online, should also be at hand for ease of reference. It is helpful to have these printed out to be provided to patients.

Metastatic Disease

Approximately 10%–15% of women with breast cancer develop distant metastases, which result in poor survival (21%). Young premenopausal women with triple-negative breast cancer (estrogen receptor, progesterone receptor, and HER2 negative) tend to have poorer outcomes (Mendoza, Moreno, & Caguioa, 2013). In a study among women with breast cancer who developed metastatic disease (Copson et al., 2013), 25.8% had spread to multiple sites including the lung (27.4%), bone (51.6%), liver (41.9%), and, less frequently, central nervous system (6.5%). Care for those with metastatic disease focuses on alleviating symptoms, maintaining quality of life, and, when possible, prolonging survival. Although the focus of care may not be on cure, participation in clinical trials may help to prolong survival.

In a United Kingdom study of women with advanced or metastatic breast cancer (Harding et al., 2013), 59% reported that they had not participated in their treatment decisions, and just 21% reported they had been informed about clinical trials. Two-thirds of the women in the study wanted access to treatment that would extend their lives so that they had time to spend with their families, and an equal proportion were willing to endure the side effects of treatment if their lives were prolonged.

For those with metastatic cancer, thoughts about the end of life must be faced. Most young adults have not experienced the death of a loved one other than an elderly grandparent or relative or the loss of friends or young family members to accidental or traumatic death. Negotiating the end of life when one's life is really only beginning is an unimaginable challenge.

End of Life

Knowledge about end-of-life care for young adults is limited, as most of the research on end-of-life care has focused on older adults, with a smaller body of knowledge in pediatric populations.

Pritchard, Cuvelier, Harlos, and Barr (2011) noted that for young adults undergoing treatment for cancer, the transition to end-of-life care often means loss of support from peers who are still in treatment and on a curative path. This results in further isolation, particularly when the young adult moves to hospice or home for end-of-life care. Younger people are more likely to die at home than in the hospital (Grinyer & Thomas, 2004), in part because their parents are more likely to want to care for them at home and are able to do so. However, not all young adults have the kind of relationship with their parents to allow this, and young adults with a partner or family of their own may not be able to be cared for in their own home and may not want to return to their parents' house for their final weeks or months of life.

In a study from France, Cohen-Gogo et al. (2011) examined the experiences of 45 adolescents and young adults with a variety of cancers (predominantly sarcoma and brain tumors). Average survival times were 18 months from diagnosis and 7 months from first relapse or signs of progression. During the last month of life, all experienced physical and psychological symptoms. The type of cancer influenced the physical symptoms experienced: those with sarcomas reported pain, dyspnea, and fatigue, whereas those with brain tumors experienced paralysis, confusion, or coma more frequently. The most frequently experienced symptoms overall were pain and dyspnea. Psychological symptoms were universal, with 100% of participants reporting sadness, anxiety, fear of being alone, fear about death and pain, and guilt. About 60% experienced nightmares, and less than 40% reported fear of treatment and anger. Forty percent of the participants in this study had received chemotherapy to alleviate symptoms during the last month of life, and one-third had received artificial nutrition during the last week of life. The authors of the study noted that administration of artificial nutrition is not unusual in the pediatric setting where these patients were treated because family members and healthcare providers perceive withdrawing nutrition as starving the patient.

How to Support the Young Adult at the End of Life

The inclusion of palliative care services into the end-of-life care plan for young adults is a sensitive topic. Healthcare providers may avoid discussing it because they do not want to be seen as "giving up" on the patient. However, this may cause a delay in appropriate end-of-life care (Pritchard et al., 2011). Palliative care is intended to alleviate suffering and control symptoms in the transition from life to death (World Health Organization, n.d.). The term *palliative care* may in itself be a barrier for inclusion of services and support by healthcare providers, parents and other family members, and the young adults themselves. A more appropriate term may be *supportive care* or *symptom management*; this may allow for earlier referral to the palliative care service or team and may help to overcome some of the barriers to acceptance (Pritchard et al., 2011). Wein, Pery, and Zer (2010) suggested that palliative care practitioners also have a role to play in facilitating care issues such as sedation, hydration and nutrition, and cessation of treatment. They also educate and support the parents to prepare them when death is inevitable and difficult decisions must be made. Challenges exist when the young adults are being treated and cared for in smaller institutions where specialized palliative care is not provided or where access is difficult because of geographic distance.

Young adults at the end of life face multiple issues, including the need for advance care planning. Multiple organizations recommend involving the patients, even younger adolescents, in planning for their care at the end of life. Advance care planning and documents allow young adults to express preferences regarding treatment if and when they cannot speak for themselves. Knowing what the patient wants is thought to be helpful to family and partners when faced with the end of life of a loved one (Wiener et al., 2012).

A number of tools can be used with young adults and their families to assist in planning for the end of life. One of the first of these was "My Thoughts, My Wishes, My Voice," developed by Aging With Dignity and containing the following eight sections.

1. The person I want to make healthcare decisions for me when I can't make them for myself
2. My wish for the kind of medical treatment I want or don't want
3. My wish for how comfortable I want to be
4. My wish for how I want people to treat me
5. My wish for what I want my loved ones to know
6. Spiritual wishes
7. How I want to be remembered
8. My voice (blank pages for writing messages for people)

This was replaced by the most recent tool, "Voicing My Choices," which was developed after a review of other advance care planning documents ("Five Wishes" and "My Thoughts, My Wishes, My Voice") (Wiener et al., 2012). This guide can be accessed at www.agingwithdignity.org/voicing-my -choices.php. It contains sections on

- Comfort measures
- Life-support measures
- Appointment of a healthcare agent
- What the person wants family and friends to know
- Spiritual thoughts and wishes
- What kind of remembrance service or funeral the person wants
- How the person's belongings are to be dealt with and shared
- Pages for messages to loved ones and friends.

"Voicing My Choices" is not a legal document and instead is a guide that allows young adults to consider what kind of care they want and what they want their friends and loved ones to know. For young adults 18 years of age and older, the recommendation is to complete the "Five Wishes" document, which is legally binding in 42 states and the District of Columbia. A sample version can be found at www.agingwithdignity.org/forms/5wishes.pdf.

"Five Wishes" contains sections on (a) naming a healthcare agent, (b) medical treatments, (c) comfort measures, and (d) additional information that loved ones should know. The use of "Five Wishes" in family-centered advance care planning was found to be feasible and allowed parents to understand and honor the wishes of their young adult child (Lyon, Jacobs, Briggs, Cheng, & Wang, 2013, 2014). The authors concluded that family-centered advance care planning is a process rather than a onetime event and allows for further discussion and revision of wishes and instructions.

Conclusion

When remission or cure does not happen, the disease takes on a new meaning. Fear of recurrence is a global phenomenon, and when cancer is diagnosed at a late stage, recurrence or metastatic disease may be a reality. Anticipating the death of a young adult is extraordinarily difficult for all involved. Children are not supposed to die before their parents, and siblings are not supposed to lose a brother or sister at a young age. This chapter has discussed the little evidence that exists about young adults facing recurrence, metastatic disease, and the end of life. Much work remains to be done in this area, both clinically and through research.

References

Bower, J.E., Woolery, A., Sternlieb, B., & Garet, D. (2005). Yoga for cancer patients and survivors. *Cancer Control, 12,* 165–171.

Cohen-Gogo, S., Marioni, G., Laurent, S., Gaspar, N., Semeraro, M., Gabolde, M., ... Brugières, L. (2011). End of life care in adolescents and young adults with cancer: Experience of the adolescent unit of the Institut Gustave Roussy. *European Journal of Cancer, 47,* 2735–2741. doi:10.1016/j.ejca.2011.09.008

Copson, E., Eccles, B., Maishman, T., Gerty, S., Stanton, L., Cutress, R.I., ... Eccles, D. (2013). Prospective observational study of breast cancer treatment outcomes for UK women aged 18–40 years at diagnosis: The POSH study. *Journal of the National Cancer Institute, 105,* 978–988. doi:10.1093/jnci/djt134

Crist, J.V., & Grunfeld, E.A. (2013). Factors reported to influence fear of recurrence in cancer patients: A systematic review. *Psycho-Oncology, 22,* 978–986. doi:10.1002/pon.3114

Filleron, T., Dalenc, F., Kramar, A., Spielmann, M., Levy, C., Fumoleau, P., ... Roché, H. (2013). Prognostic factors of young women (≤ 35 years) with node positive breast cancer: Possible influence on post-therapeutic follow-up. *Bulletin du Cancer, 100*(7–8), 22–29. doi:10.1684/bdc.2013.1791

Gil, K.M., Mishel, M.H., Belyea, M., Germino, B., Porter, L.S., LaNey, I.C., & Stewart, J. (2004). Triggers of uncertainty about recurrence and long-term treatment effects in older African American and Caucasian breast cancer survivors. *Oncology Nursing Forum, 31,* 633–639. doi:10.1188/04.ONF.633-639

Grinyer, A., & Thomas, C. (2004). The importance of place of death in young adults with terminal cancer. *Mortality, 9,* 114–131. doi:10.1080/13576270310001659436

Harding, V., Afshar, M., Krell, J., Ramaswami, R., Twelves, C.J., & Stebbing, J. (2013). "Being there" for women with metastatic breast cancer: A pan-European patient survey. *British Journal of Cancer, 109,* 1543–1548. doi:10.1038/bjc.2013.492

Liukkonen, S., Leidenius, M., Saarto, T., & Sjöström-Mattson, J. (2011). Breast cancer in very young women. *European Journal of Surgical Oncology, 37,* 1030–1037. doi:10.1016/j.ejso.2011.08.133

Lyon, M.E., Jacobs, S., Briggs, L., Cheng, Y.I., & Wang, J. (2013). Family-centered advance care planning for teens with cancer. *JAMA Pediatrics, 167,* 460–467. doi:10.1001/jamapediatrics.2013.943

Lyon, M.E., Jacobs, S., Briggs, L., Cheng, Y.I., & Wang, J. (2014). A longitudinal, randomized, controlled trial of advance care planning for teens with cancer: Anxiety, depression, quality of life, advance directives, spirituality. *Journal of Adolescent Health, 54,* 710–717. doi:10.1016/j.jadohealth.2013.10.206

Mendoza, E.S.R., Moreno, E., & Caguioa, P.B. (2013). Predictors of early distant metastasis in women with breast cancer. *Journal of Cancer Research and Clinical Oncology, 139,* 645–652. doi:10.1007/s00432-012-1367-z

Miles, A., Simon, A., & Wardle, J. (2010). Answering patient questions about the role lifestyle factors play in cancer onset and recurrence: What do health care professionals say? *Journal of Health Psychology, 15,* 291–298. doi:10.1177/1359105309351245

Osborn, R.L., Demoncada, A.C., & Feuerstein, M. (2006). Psychosocial interventions for depression, anxiety, and quality of life in cancer survivors: Meta-analyses. *International Journal of Psychiatry in Medicine, 36,* 13–34. doi:10.2190/EUFN-RV1K-Y3TR-FK0L

Pritchard, S., Cuvelier, G., Harlos, M., & Barr, R. (2011). Palliative care in adolescents and young adults with cancer. *Cancer, 117*(Suppl. 10), 2323–2328. doi:10.1002/cncr.26044

Simard, S., Savard, S., & Ivers, H. (2010). Fear of cancer recurrence: Specific profiles and nature of intrusive thoughts. *Journal of Cancer Survivorship, 4,* 261–271. doi:10.1007/s11764-010-0136-8

Siponen, E.T., Joensuu, H., & Leidenius, M.H.K. (2013). Local recurrence of breast cancer after mastectomy and modern multidisciplinary treatment. *Acta Oncologica, 52,* 66–72. doi:10.3109/0284186X.2012.718793

Steele, N., Haigh, R., Knowles, G., & Mckean, M. (2007). Carcinoembryonic antigen (CEA) testing in colorectal cancer follow up: What do patients think? *Postgraduate Medicine, 83,* 612–614. doi:10.1136/pgmj.2007.059634

Thewes, B., Brebach, R., Dzidowska, M., Rhodes, P., Sharpe, L., & Butow, P. (2014). Current approaches to managing fear of cancer recurrence; a descriptive survey of psychosocial and clinical health professionals. *Psycho-Oncology, 23,* 390–396. doi:10.1002/pon.3423

Thewes, B., Butow, P., Bell, M.L., Beith, J., Stuart-Harris, R., Grossi, M., … FCR Study Advisory Committee. (2012). Fear of cancer recurrence in young women with a history of early-stage breast cancer: A cross-sectional study of prevalence and association with health behaviours. *Supportive Care in Cancer, 20,* 2651–2659. doi:10.1007/s00520-011-1371-x

Tichy, J.R., Lim, E., & Anders, C.K. (2013). Breast cancer in adolescents and young adults: A review with a focus on biology. *Journal of the National Comprehensive Cancer Network, 11,* 1060–1069. Retrieved from http://www.jnccn.org/content/11/9/1060.long

Todd, B.L., Moskowitz, M.C., Ottati, A., & Feuerstein, M. (2014). Stressors, stress response, and cancer recurrence: A systematic review. *Cancer Nursing, 37,* 114–125. doi:10.1097/NCC.0b013e318289a6e2

Vivar, C.G., Canga, N., Canga, A.D., & Arantzamendi, M. (2009). The psychosocial impact of recurrence on cancer survivors and family members: A narrative review. *Journal of Advanced Nursing, 65,* 724–736. doi:10.1111/j.1365-2648.2008.04939.x

Wein, S., Pery, S., & Zer, A. (2010). Role of palliative care in adolescent and young adult oncology. *Journal of Clinical Oncology, 28,* 4819–4824. doi:10.1200/JCO.2009.22.4543

Wiener, L., Zadeh, S., Battles, H., Baird, K., Ballard, E., Osherow, J., & Pao, M. (2012). Allowing adolescents and young adults to plan their end-of-life care. *Pediatrics, 130,* 897–905. doi:10.1542/peds.2012-0663

World Health Organization. (n.d.). WHO definition of palliative care. Retrieved from http://www.who.int/cancer/palliative/definition/en

CHAPTER 13
Disease-Specific Concerns

Introduction

This book contains many examples of how breast and gynecologic cancers affect young adults because this is where most of the research has been conducted. However, other cancers—for example, testicular, colorectal, hematologic, and thyroid—also affect young adults. Genetic mutations, particularly *BRCA1* and *BRCA2*, also deserve attention because of the impact of increased risk for breast and ovarian cancer in young women who carry the mutation(s).

This chapter is intended to provide a brief overview of these topics. Additional information also can be found in the chapters on sexuality and fertility (Chapters 5 and 6).

Testicular Cancer

Testicular cancer is the most common solid tumor in young adult men. It is highly curable, with a mean 10-year survival rate of 95% (Hanna & Einhorn, 2014). Because of the young age at diagnosis, survivors of this cancer live for many years and thus are at risk for long-term and late effects of the cancer, including the risk of developing a second cancer, often leukemia, which is treatment related. Long-term effects include the development of metabolic syndrome, cardiovascular disease, damage to the lungs and kidneys depending on the chemotherapy agents used, hypogonadism, and infertility, in addition to psychosocial effects (Hanna & Einhorn, 2014). Because this cancer involves the testicle, it has unique challenges for the young adult male that may influence his life like no other cancer. The sexual side effects of being diagnosed with and treated for testicular cancer are described in detail in Chapter 5.

In a study of 21 young adult survivors of testicular cancer, participants described the experience of the disease and its impact on life after cancer

(Carpentier & Fortenberry, 2010). Embarrassment led to delays in seeking help, and it was often their partner who forced them into seeking medical attention. After the diagnosis, the young men reported that they felt different from everyone else. The young men in this study described themselves as "damaged goods"; hair loss, surgical scars, and the loss of a testicle led to issues related to masculine identity. Many felt vulnerable, in part related to the risk of the cancer recurring in the other testicle. Another concern was that of disclosure about the cancer. For men who were not partnered, deciding when to tell a potential partner was a concern, and some had avoided romantic relationships because of this. Some of the young men also were concerned about disclosing the diagnosis to their male friends, many of whom joked about it. On the other hand, some survivors chose to play an advocacy role and encouraged others to perform testicular self-examination.

These young men have unmet needs for information too. In a study from the Netherlands that surveyed 264 testicular cancer survivors (Jonker-Pool et al., 2004), 53% reported having insufficient information, and 54% reported receiving insufficient support during treatment. Two-thirds of the sample needed information during follow-up, and 29.5% reported one or more sexual problems after treatment. An Australian study (Smith et al., 2013) suggested that unmet needs for supportive care are related to the development of anxiety and depression in testicular cancer survivors, and in turn, these are related to poor health-related quality of life. In this study of 244 testicular cancer survivors, 66% reported one or more unmet needs. The most common unmet needs were related to fear of recurrence, sexual problems, and life stress.

Testicular cancer has an impact on quality of life. In a study of men in the military with testicular cancer (Kim et al., 2011), chemotherapy conferred additional quality-of-life risks with a trend toward poorer mental health and impaired social functioning in those treated with chemotherapy. In another study, Skaali et al. (2011) found that smoking and alcohol use were associated with cancer-related distress in newly diagnosed men with testicular cancer.

The impact of testicular cancer on fertility is an important issue in survivorship. Many men diagnosed with testicular cancer have poor sperm counts or motility before treatment (Liguori et al., 2008). This may be related to multiple factors, including undescended testes in childhood, hormone production by the tumor, or stress related to the diagnosis. The value of sperm banking for these men cannot be emphasized enough; however, long-term fertility is not necessarily destroyed in all men treated for this cancer. In one study (Molnár et al., 2014), 22% of the men reported unassisted pregnancies in their partners four years after treatment. Close to 12% of the men in this study had used frozen sperm to conceive, and of these, 57% of their partners had a live birth. In another study, 49.3%

of men treated with surgery were able to father children (Matos, Škrbinc, & Zakotnik, 2010). Magelssen et al. (2005) reported that although 50% of their patients were interested in sperm banking before treatment, only 7% of patients used the frozen sperm. They concluded that the financial costs of assisted reproductive technology might have played a role in the low rate. Seventeen percent of their sample fathered at least one child after treatment. In an American study (Kim et al., 2010), distress related to fertility was thought to be caused by the mention of infertility after treatment. However, in this study, testicular cancer survivors were as likely to father children as the control group.

Young men face a number of struggles because of their gender. Cancer is experienced as a biographical disruption and interferes with the way people make sense of the world around them and their own selves. Cancer challenges them with uncertainty within the context of a discordant and troubled future. They experience isolation from their peers and colleagues and struggle with their experience of illness within societal views of the male body (Wenger, 2013a). Campbell-Enns and Woodgate (2013) reviewed the literature on young men with cancer and identified the following themes: having cancer calls into question the traditional views on manhood; fatherhood was a struggle, as men may not be able to fulfill their roles as protector and provider; family bonds, both with parents and their own children, are important; communicating about the cancer is very difficult and cancer talk is often silenced; and men live with uncertainty and struggle to cope with this uncertainty. Wenger (2013b) theorized that men with cancer cope not only by having a strong back that allows them to build resources that minimize the shift in their lives as a result of the cancer, but also by having a soft front that allows them to seek help so that they can adapt to the disruption in their lives from cancer.

How to Help the Young Adult With Testicular Cancer

Because testicular cancer affects an important part of masculinity and sexuality, it is very important for healthcare providers to be sensitive to the distress that a young man is experiencing, even if he does not openly discuss or even show this. The diagnosis and treatment of testicular cancer are shocking and fear provoking for many young men, not just because cancer itself is unexpected at a young age, but also because of the need for frequent exposure of a private body part. Acknowledgment of this can help patients to open up and discuss what they are feeling or break down some of the walls they may have built up as a coping mechanism.

Young men may not disclose their innermost feelings to their friends. Thus, referral to a support group of other young adult men may be a lifeline. Supportive care is discussed in greater detail in Chapter 9.

BRCA1 and *BRCA2* Mutation Carriers

The most well-known genetic risk factors for cancer are the *BRCA1* and *BRCA2* gene mutations that are involved with the development of hereditary breast and ovarian cancer (HBOC). The risk of developing breast or ovarian cancer before the age of 30 is low (3.4% for *BRCA1* and 1.5% for *BRCA2* for breast cancer and 1%–2% for ovarian cancer [either *BRCA1* or *BRCA2*]) (Chen et al., 2006; Chen & Parmigiani, 2007). These may appear to be high relative risks, but the absolute risk is low: 95% of women younger than age 30 with the mutation will not develop breast or ovarian cancer (Hoskins, Werner-Lin, & Greene, 2014).

However, the knowledge of mutation carrier status changes the life of young women in many ways. Few evidence-based guidelines exist for the management of risk for young women with the mutation. Options include surveillance with regular mammograms and clinical and self-breast examination, blood tests for the presence of CA 125 (a marker of ovarian cancer that is not a screening test), chemoprevention with tamoxifen to prevent breast cancer or oral contraceptives to lower the risk of ovarian cancer, and risk-reducing surgery, such as prophylactic bilateral mastectomy or bilateral salpingo-oophorectomy (Hoskins, Roy, & Greene, 2012). All of these strategies have side effects that will profoundly affect quality of life, including anxiety about repeated screening and waiting for test results, side effects of medications, altered body image, the need for early childbearing, or infertility.

For many women, merely knowing their *BRCA1* or *BRCA2* carrier status is shocking, and their perception is often framed within the experience of a family member's (usually the woman's mother) breast cancer. Researchers have found that for some women, family narratives of risk are more influential than the facts of absolute risk (Hoskins et al., 2012). In this study, young women reported that the information understood during the genetic testing process formed the basis of their understanding of personal risk. Healthcare providers may intensify the perception of risk for young women and lead them to believe their risk is high and their health precarious. This may cause women to make rushed and uncertain decisions about risk management that are based not on fact but rather fear of the unknown (Hoskins et al., 2014). This study showed that many young women have poor health literacy and that the complex nature of risk discussion was confusing. Many overestimated their risk of cancer, seemingly ignoring short-term risk for the more serious lifetime risk and also focusing on relative rather than absolute risk. Many young women have limited experience making life-altering decisions, and being single and childless has additional implications for deciding about risk management in this context (Hamilton & Hurley, 2010).

Young women frequently ask their parents for help in navigating this complex situation emotionally, logistically, and financially. Werner-Lin, Hoskins, Doyle, and Greene (2012) reported that in some instances, women agreed to genetic testing to ease parental anxiety or because their parent or parents asked them to. In this study, all the participants consulted with the parent's healthcare providers, resulting in situations where privacy and autonomy were compromised. In some instances, the young women saw the healthcare provider with the parent present, leading to silencing and reluctance to ask questions or seek clarification of the information provided in an attempt to protect the parent from upset. In some cases, the healthcare provider disclosed confidential information about the young adult's mutation status to the parent first, an obvious transgression of privacy and confidentiality rights. The financial and emotional dependence of the young woman may limit her ability to make decisions independently, and this can have far-reaching effects on her life (Hoskins & Werner-Lin, 2013). For these reasons, access to an independent genetic counselor for education and decision making is vitally important.

Risk management options for young women who carry the genetic mutation for HBOC are different than for older women who have completed their families. Surveillance with regular and repeated examinations and screening tests are onerous, expensive, and often fear provoking. In one study, participants viewed surveillance as waiting for cancer rather than preventing cancer (Hoskins & Greene, 2012). For many young women, the ability to continue with surveillance depends on how long they can tolerate the stress of screening. Suspicious findings on mammograms and magnetic resonance imaging resulted in biopsies, and the resultant anxiety for many led to a decision to have risk-reducing surgery, even for those who were young and had not yet started childbearing.

Related to this is many people's belief that cancer is inevitable. Their experience of a family member's cancer and their desire to avoid the same suffering, both personally and by the family, creates an urgency to have risk-reducing surgery. For some, the urgency is compounded by a desire to have bilateral mastectomies *before* settling down with a life partner and having children (Hoskins & Greene, 2012). Some women choose to have bilateral prophylactic mastectomy first, followed by salpingo-oophorectomy when they have completed their families. This can lead to losses related to the inability to breast-feed; however, all women must weigh the risks and benefits of early surgical intervention. Their decision may be influenced by fears of cancer developing while they are pregnant and unable to have mammograms and other screening tests.

Deciding about surgery is difficult, and young women seek advice from healthcare providers, family and friends, and the larger breast cancer community (Klitzman & Chung, 2009). Women in the study by Klitzman and Chung (2009) struggled with whether to have surgery and when to have it. They then had to consider the side effects of surgery and the potential impact on body image and sexuality, as well as on romantic relationships. When consulting physicians about their choices, women in this study wanted clear and unambiguous opinions. They did not always receive this; some physicians were not directive, which led to dissatisfaction on the part of patients who wanted recommendations. Others found that the advice from their physician was too honest, and both the content and the tone created additional stress in an already stressful situation. Asking family and friends for advice had the same potential for conflicting opinions. However, the participants reported supportive and reinforcing relationships as being very helpful. Finally, those who sought support and information from both online and face-to-face interactions with women in breast cancer communities found connecting with those who had been through similar experiences was highly beneficial; although for some, the information was scary and upsetting (Klitzman & Chung, 2009).

The consequences of risk-reducing surgery are far reaching. Hamilton and Hurley (2010) reported on a sample of young women who identified three distinct experiences: challenges related to dating, the risks to relationships from disclosure, and the impact of surgery and treatment for breast cancer. The young women in this study described challenges similar to those discussed in Chapter 4. When and how to disclose their genetic status or altered body after mastectomy caused the women anxiety in addition to fears of potential rejection. They also reported a sense of urgency to have children once they were in a relationship. This, in turn, influenced the pace of the relationship. This was especially challenging when considering how long they had been in the relationship, and a small minority of the women in this study had experienced a breakup after learning about their positive mutation status. The impact of surgery and treatment was experienced as a sense of loss. The losses were real—removal of breasts—and also potential—loss of fertility. However, for some, a prophylactic mastectomy reflected a loss of worry about developing breast cancer later in life.

How to Help the Young Adult Who Carries a Genetic Mutation

It is never clear how a young woman will respond to the news that she carries the *BRCA* gene mutation. For that reason, it is imperative that she receive appropriate counseling both before and after the test. Counseling before the test is important because if she understands the consequences, she may delay screening until she has achieved certain milestones, or she may agree to the screening but have a better understanding of the choices that she has in terms of future actions. It also is important that she have counseling without a parent present, which may be the most challenging aspect of all. Sharing a healthcare provider with a parent may be good for understanding family history and dynamics, but multiple challenges arise from the emotions present when a mother carries the genes for HBOC and the daughter has questions or concerns about her health and her options related to screening. It is much better for the young woman to have counseling alone and from a qualified professional who does not have a relationship with her parent and who is an expert in the intricacies of genetic testing.

In addition, healthcare providers who see young women at risk for HBOC should not pressure them to have children urgently. This may force them into relationships that are not right for them and potentially exposes them to rejection when they tell a prospective partner about their status. Having children is a big step, and feeling pressure to conceive will complicate their relationship choices. It also is important to be aware that young adult women at increased risk for HBOC may feel isolated from and out of sync with their peers who do not have the same pressures to have children or undergo major surgery. It is important to offer support over time and within the context of each young woman's life. They may only receive helpful support from those who are going through the same experience, so referral to support groups and websites may be the best that healthcare providers can offer these women.

The following websites may be helpful to those who carry *BRCA* mutations.
* Bright Pink: www.bebrightpink.org
* FORCE (Facing Our Risk of Cancer Empowered): www.facingourrisk.org
* Susan G. Komen: ww5.komen.org/BreastCancer/InheritedGeneticMutations .html
* Young Survival Coalition: www.youngsurvival.org

Hematologic Cancers

Hematologic cancers, including acute lymphoblastic leukemia, acute myeloid leukemia, and lymphoma, occur frequently in young adults. With improved treatments, it is now possible for individuals to live much longer, and a portion ultimately survive what was previously a terminal cancer (Mattson, Demshar, & Daly, 2013). However, almost no research exists on the experience of these individuals other than descriptions of the multimodality treatments, including bone marrow or stem cell transplants, they receive.

Pidala, Anasetti, and Jim (2009) stated that individuals undergoing hematopoietic cell transplantation (HCT) need to know that the procedure is arduous and causes numerous side effects that potentially affect quality of life; 25% will experience ongoing medical and emotional challenges. However, they also stated that more than 60% of transplant recipients report good quality of life within one to two years after the transplant. Depression and distress are described as long-term side effects after transplantation, along with fatigue, insomnia, and relationship problems (Majhail et al., 2012). Graft-versus-host disease often has skin and mucous membrane manifestations that can affect sexual functioning, adding to distress.

In a study of transplant recipients with a mean age of 43 (Pillay, Lee, Katona, Burney, & Avery, 2014), 15% experienced distress at about a year following transplant. Being single and having physical side effects were associated with poorer survival. However, it is not clear if the results of this study are applicable to the young adult population. In their review of long-term survivors of HCT, Syrjala, Martin, and Lee (2012) noted that survivors are resilient and cope well with the transplant and survivorship. However, the authors acknowledged that the emotional demands of life after HCT are challenging and include fear of recurrence, uncertainty, anxiety about follow-up testing, hypervigilance, depression, anger, and post-traumatic stress. They also noted that 90% of survivors report post-traumatic growth and a greater appreciation of life. In a review of studies of unmet needs of individuals with hematologic cancer, once again not restricted to young adults, the most prevalent unmet needs identified were fear of recurrence and issues related to fertility (Swash, Hulbert-Williams, & Bramwell, 2014).

The only study of quality of life in young adults (Mattson et al., 2013) reported that 69% of the participants (N = 48) were worried about the cancer recurring. Other issues affecting quality of life included moving on and returning to "normal" life and dealing with long-term side effects, fatigue, changes in social relationships, and financial or employment problems. When participants were asked what would have been helpful after the transplant, 44% stated that nothing would have helped, 25% stated that support groups would be helpful, and 19% of the survivors indicated wanting more information and education about what to expect.

How to Help the Young Adult With Hematologic Cancer

Given the understanding of the seriousness of the diagnosis at a young age as well as the challenges of multimodal treatment or transplantation, it is imperative that healthcare providers screen for depression and distress regularly in these young survivors. Majhail et al. (2012) suggested routine screening every 6–12 months, including sexual health assessment. They also recommended providing young survivors with clear education and advice about contraception and fertility.

It is important to assess for and treat graft-versus-host disease aggressively because it can affect sexual functioning and cause further distress related to altered relationships. Many young survivors of hematologic cancers are given the message, overtly or covertly, that after going through what they have, they should just be happy to be alive. This is harmful and alienating.

Healthcare providers need to encourage these survivors to instead live life fully, given what they have gone through and survived.

Colorectal Cancer

Colorectal cancer is rare in young adults, but the incidence is increasing (Ahnen et al., 2014). Although screening is not recommended for those younger than age 50, young adults with familial syndromes are known to be at significantly higher risk and should have regular testing for the presence of polyps (Ahnen et al., 2014). Young adults typically present with later-stage disease and tend to develop distant recurrence over time (You et al., 2011). They also are more likely to die of their disease (Forbes et al., 2010).

Because colorectal cancer is rare in young adults, it is thought that all newly diagnosed patients should be seen by a medical oncologist, even where the protocol is for patients in this age group to receive care from a pediatric oncologist. This is because medical oncologists have greater experience treating this cancer and will be able to develop an aggressive treatment plan (Goldberg & Furman, 2012). Advances in the treatment of colorectal cancer have occurred, with new chemotherapies that show survival benefits and biologic agents for the treatment of metastatic disease (Zbuk, Sidebotham, Bleyer, & La Quaglia, 2009).

Young adults with colorectal cancer experience a significant symptom burden including pain, fatigue, nausea, dyspnea, drowsiness, and distress. These symptoms interfere with multiple aspects of daily life including activities of normal life, relationships, ability to work or attend school or college, mood, and general enjoyment of life (Sanford et al., 2014).

How to Help the Young Adult With Colorectal Cancer

Young adults with colorectal cancer carry a significant burden of disease and treatment, and no data-driven evidence exists in the literature about interventions for this population. Given the nature of the disease and the involvement of private body parts in both diagnosis and treatment, these individuals will likely experience real and perceived invasion of private body parts with repeated rectal examinations, as well as surgery resulting in an ostomy (temporary or permanent). These can all have a severe impact on body image and self-esteem. Many young adults are diagnosed with late-stage disease, which has existential implications.

Chapter 5 contains a detailed discussion about the sexual effects from colorectal cancer treatment. Because of the proximity of the colon to reproductive organs, surgery and radiation may affect fertility. In a case report, surgeons transposed the ovaries of five women prior to radiation for rectal cancer. They also performed an ovarian wedge resection to preserve ovarian tissue. One of the patients subsequently gave birth to a healthy baby girl (Elizur et al., 2009). Spanos and Mamopoulos (2010) suggested that all young women with rectal cancer be informed about the risks of treatment for future fertility, given the experimental nature of these fertility-preservation techniques.

Thyroid Cancer

Although still relatively low, the incidence of thyroid cancers in young adults is rising, with many more young women being diagnosed than men (Vergamini, Frazier, Abrantes, Ribeiro, & Rodriguez-Galindo, 2014). Most people will be treated with surgery to remove the gland as well as radioactive iodine and will require replacement thyroid hormone therapy for the rest of their lives. External beam radiation therapy to the area typically is used only in cases of recurrence or to treat metastatic disease. Side effects of treatment include dry mouth, the potential for hoarseness if damage to the nerves supplying the vocal cords occurred during surgery, memory problems, and fatigue (Ying, Huh, Bottomley, Evans, & Waguespack, 2009).

The potential for significant psychosocial side effects exists despite, or perhaps because of, the high cure rate. Easley, Miedema, and Robinson (2013) interviewed 12 young adult survivors with thyroid cancer, and their descriptions of the experience and subsequent psychosocial outcomes are illuminating. The survivors described that the seriousness of the diagnosis was largely ignored—it is the "good cancer"—and that because they did not experience the common side effects of chemotherapy such as hair loss, support for what they were going through was largely absent. They noted that although thyroid cancer may not be life threatening, it is still a cancer diagnosis and is life altering. They described the isolation they felt after receiving radioactive iodine, as they had to remain alone in a room to avoid exposing others to the high radiation doses they had ingested. Some said that they felt like zoo animals or as if they had the plague when they were in hospital after this treatment. They talked about feeling isolated from other cancer survivors because their experience was viewed as being much "easier" than chemotherapy, so other survivors did not want to talk to them about their cancer experience.

How to Help the Young Adult With Thyroid Cancer

Given the sense of isolation experienced by thyroid cancer survivors (Easley et al., 2013), it is imperative that oncology care providers temper the hope from a relatively nonlethal cancer with acknowledgment that any cancer is life altering for those who are diagnosed. For healthcare providers, being aware of the language used when talking about this cancer is the first step. Although it is important to give patients accurate information about statistics, including mortality, it is also important to avoid making patients feel unimportant when compared to others who have more advanced disease or life-threatening cancers.

Supporting young adults with thyroid cancer is important because their experience is isolating and frightening, and despite good outcomes, they may experience the same fears of recurrence and distress as others with more "serious" cancers. It may be challenging to find an in-person support group of only thyroid cancer survivors in most cities, so online support groups may be very helpful for these young adults because they are more likely to find others across the country (or world) who can relate to their unique experiences.

Conclusion

This chapter has described the challenges of some of the other cancers affecting young adults, as the majority of research, and therefore much of this book, has focused on women with breast cancer. Greater detail about psychosocial effects can be found in the chapters dedicated to sexuality, fertility, distress, and supportive care.

References

Ahnen, D.J., Wade, S.W., Jones, W.F., Sifri, R., Silveiras, J.M., Greenamyer, J., ... You, Y.N. (2014). The increasing incidence of young-onset colorectal cancer: A call to action. *Mayo Clinic Proceedings, 89,* 216–224. doi:10.1016/j.mayocp.2013.09.006

Campbell-Enns, H.J., & Woodgate, R.L. (2013). Young men with cancer: A literature review. *Cancer Nursing, 36,* E36–E47. doi:10.1097/NCC.0b013e31824e8c58

Carpentier, M.Y., & Fortenberry, J.D. (2010). Romantic and sexual relationships, body image, and fertility in adolescent and young adult testicular cancer survivors: A review of the literature. *Journal of Adolescent Health, 47,* 115–125. doi:10.1016/j.jadohealth.2010.04.005

Chen, S., Iversen, E., Friebel, T., Finkelstein, D., Weber, B.L., Eisen, A., ... Parmigiani, G. (2006). Characterization of *BRCA1* and *BRCA2* mutations in a large United States sample. *Journal of Clinical Oncology, 24,* 863–871. doi:10.1200/JCO.2005.03.6772

Chen, S., & Parmigiani, G. (2007). Meta-analysis of *BRCA1* and *BRCA2* penetrance. *Journal of Clinical Oncology, 25,* 1329–1333. doi:10.1200/JCO.2006.09.1066

Easley, J., Miedema, B., & Robinson, L. (2013). It's the "good" cancer, so who cares? Perceived lack of support among young thyroid cancer survivors. *Oncology Nursing Forum, 40,* 596–600. doi:10.1188/13.ONF.596-600

Elizur, S.E., Tulandi, T., Meterissian, S., Huang, J.Y.J., Levin, D., & Tan, S.L. (2009). Fertility preservation for young women with rectal cancer—A combined approach from one referral center. *Journal of Gastrointestinal Surgery, 13,* 1111–1115. doi:10.1007/s11605-009-0829-3

Forbes, S.S., Sutradhar, R., Paszat, L.F., Rabeneck, L., Urbach, D.R., & Baxter, N.N. (2010). Long-term survival in young adults with colorectal cancer: A population-based study. *Diseases of the Colon and Rectum, 53,* 973–978. doi:10.1007/DCR.0b013e3181cf8341

Goldberg, J., & Furman, W.L. (2012). Management of colorectal carcinoma in children and young adults. *Journal of Pediatric Hematology/Oncology, 34*(Suppl. 2), S76–S79. doi:10.1097/MPH.0b013e31824e38c1

Hamilton, R., & Hurley, K.E. (2010). Conditions and consequences of a *BRCA* mutation in young, single women of childbearing age. *Oncology Nursing Forum, 37,* 627–634. doi:10.1188/10.ONF.627-634

Hanna, N., & Einhorn, L.H. (2014). Testicular cancer: A reflection on 50 years of discovery. *Journal of Clinical Oncology, 32,* 3085–3092. doi:10.1200/JCO.2014.56.0896

Hoskins, L.M., & Greene, M.H. (2012). Anticipatory loss and early mastectomy for young female BRCA1/2 mutation carriers. *Qualitative Health Research, 22,* 1633–1646. doi:10.1177/1049732312458182

Hoskins, L.M., Roy, K.M., & Greene, M.H. (2012). Toward a new understanding of risk perception among young female *BRCA1/2* "previvors." *Families, Systems, and Health, 30,* 32–46. doi:10.1037/a0027276

Hoskins, L.M., & Werner-Lin, A. (2013). A multi-case report of the pathways to and through genetic testing and cancer risk management for *BRCA* mutation-positive women aged 18–25. *Journal of Genetic Counseling, 22,* 27–38. doi:10.1007/s10897-012-9521-y

Hoskins, L.M., Werner-Lin, A., & Greene, M.H. (2014). In their own words: Treating very young *BRCA1/2* mutation-positive women with care and caution. *PLOS ONE, 9,* e87696. doi:10.1371/journal.pone.0087696

Jonker-Pool, G., Hoekstra, H.J., van Imhoff, G.W., Sonneveld, D.J.A., Sleijfer, D.T., van Driel, M.F., ... van de Wiel, H.B.M. (2004). Male sexuality after cancer treatment—Needs for information and support: Testicular cancer compared to malignant lymphoma. *Patient Education and Counseling, 52,* 143–150. doi:10.1016/S0738-3991(03)00025-9

Kim, C., McGlynn, K.A., McCorkle, R., Erickson, R.L., Niebuhr, D.W., Ma, S., ... Zhang, Y. (2011). Quality of life among testicular cancer survivors: A case-control study in the United States. *Quality of Life Research, 20,* 1629–1637. doi:10.1007/s11136-011-9907-6

Kim, C., McGlynn, K.A., McCorkle, R., Zheng, T., Erickson, R.L., Niebuhr, D.W., ... Zhang, Y. (2010). Fertility among testicular cancer survivors: A case-control study in the U.S. *Journal of Cancer Survivorship, 4,* 266–273. doi:10.1007/s11764-010-0134-x

Klitzman, R., & Chung, W. (2009). The process of deciding about prophylactic surgery for breast and ovarian cancer: Patient questions, uncertainties, and communication. *American Journal of Medical Genetics, 152A,* 52–66. doi:10.1002/ajmg.a.33068

Liguori, G., Trombetta, C., Bucci, S., Benvenuto, S., Amodeo, A., Ocello, G., & Belgrano, E. (2008). Semen quality before and after orchiectomy in men with testicular cancer. *Archivio Italiano di Urologia, Andrologia, 80,* 99–102.

Magelssen, H., Haugen, T.B., von Düring, V., Melve, K.K., Sandstad, B., & Fosså, S.D. (2005). Twenty years experience with semen cryopreservation in testicular cancer patients: Who needs it? *European Urology, 48,* 779–785. doi:10.1016/j.eururo.2005.05.002

Majhail, N.S., Rizzo, J.D., Lee, S.J., Aljurf, M., Atsuta, Y., Bonfim, C., ... Tichelli, A. (2012). Recommended screening and preventive practices for long-term survivors after hematopoietic cell transplantation. *Revista Brasileira de Hematologia e Hemoterapia, 34,* 109–133. Retrieved from http://www.ncbi.nlm.nih.gov/pmc/articles/PMC3459383

Matos, E., Škrbinc, B., & Zakotnik, B. (2010). Fertility in patients treated for testicular cancer. *Journal of Cancer Survivorship, 4,* 274–278. doi:10.1007/s11764-010-0135-9

Mattson, M.R., Demshar, R.K., & Daly, B.J. (2013). Quality of life of young adult survivors of hematologic malignancies. *Cancer Nursing, 36*(2), E1–E7. doi:10.1097/NCC.0b013e31824242dd

Molnár, Z., Berta, E., Benyó, M., Póka, R., Kassai, Z., Flaskó, T., ... Bodor, M. (2014). Fertility of testicular cancer patients after anticancer treatment—Experience of 11 years. *Die Pharmazie, 69,* 437–441.

Pidala, J., Anasetti, C., & Jim, H. (2009). Quality of life after allogeneic hematopoietic cell transplantation. *Blood, 114,* 7–19. doi:10.1182/blood-2008-10-182592

Pillay, B., Lee, S.J., Katona, L., Burney, S., & Avery, S. (2014). Psychosocial factors predicting survival after allogeneic stem cell transplant. *Supportive Care in Cancer, 22,* 2547–2555. doi:10.1007/s00520-014-2239-7

Sanford, S.D., Zhao, F., Salsman, J.M., Chang, V.T., Wagner, L.I., & Fisch, M.J. (2014). Symptom burden among young adults with breast or colon cancer. *Cancer, 120,* 2255–2263. doi:10.1002/cncr.28297

Skaali, T., Fosså, S.D., Andersson, S., Langberg, C.W., Lehne, G., & Dahl, A.A. (2011). Is psychological distress in men recently diagnosed with testicular cancer associated with their neuropsychological test performance? *Psycho-Oncology, 20,* 369–377. doi:10.1002/pon.1737

Smith, A., King, M., Butow, P., Luckett, T., Grimison, P., Toner, G.C., ... Olver, I. (2013). The prevalence and correlates of supportive care needs in testicular cancer survivors: A cross-sectional study. *Psycho-Oncology, 22,* 2557–2564. doi:10.1002/pon.3323

Spanos, C.P., & Mamopoulos, A. (2010). Fertility preservation for young women with rectal cancer—A combined approach from one referral center [Letter to the editor]. *Journal of Gastrointestinal Surgery, 14,* 1476. doi:10.1007/s11605-010-1271-2

Swash, B., Hulbert-Williams, N., & Bramwell, R. (2014). Unmet psychosocial needs in haematological cancer: A systematic review. *Supportive Care in Cancer, 22,* 1131–1141. doi:10.1007/s00520-014-2123-5

Syrjala, K.L., Martin, P.J., & Lee, S.J. (2012). Delivering care to long-term adult survivors of hematopoietic cell transplantation. *Journal of Clinical Oncology, 30,* 3746–3751. doi:10.1200/JCO.2012.42.3038

Vergamini, L.B., Frazier, A.L., Abrantes, F.L., Ribeiro, K.B., & Rodriguez-Galindo, C. (2014). Increase in the incidence of differentiated thyroid carcinoma in children, adolescents, and young adults: A population-based study. *Journal of Pediatrics, 164,* 1481–1485. doi:10.1016/j.jpeds.2014.01.059

Wenger, L.M. (2013a). "Living under assault": Men making sense of cancer. *European Journal of Cancer Care, 22,* 389–399. doi:10.1111/ecc.12042

Wenger, L.M. (2013b). Moving through illness with strong backs and soft fronts: A substantive theory of men's help-seeking during cancer. *Men and Masculinities, 16,* 517–539. doi:10.1177/1097184X13501177

Werner-Lin, A., Hoskins, L.M., Doyle, M.H., & Greene, M.H. (2012). "Cancer doesn't have an age": Genetic testing and cancer risk management in *BRCA1/2* mutation-positive women aged 18–24. *Health, 16,* 636–654. doi:10.1177/1363459312442420

Ying, A.K., Huh, W., Bottomley, S., Evans, D.B., & Waguespack, S.G. (2009). Thyroid cancer in young adults. *Seminars in Oncology, 36,* 258–274. doi:10.1053/j.seminoncol.2009.03.009

You, Y.N., Dozois, E.J., Boardman, L.A., Aakre, J., Huebner, M., & Larson, D.W. (2011). Young-onset rectal cancer: Presentation, pattern of care and long-term oncologic outcomes compared to a matched older-onset cohort. *Annals of Surgical Oncology, 18,* 2469–2476. doi:10.1245/s10434-011-1674-7

Zbuk, K., Sidebotham, E.L., Bleyer, A., & La Quaglia, M.P. (2009). Colorectal cancer in young adults. *Seminars in Oncology, 36,* 439–450. doi:10.1053/j.seminoncol.2009.07.008

Index

The letter f after a page number indicates that relevant content appears in a figure; the letter t, in a table.

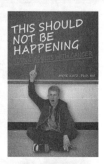
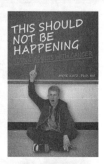
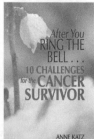
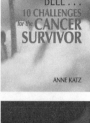
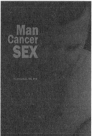
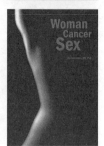